Supernatural Childbirth

40-Week Pregnancy Journal

Jackie Mize
with Terry Mize

Supernatural Childbirth

40-Week Pregnancy Journal

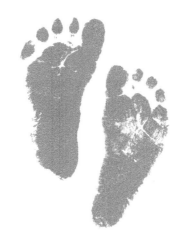

Experiencing the Promise of God for Your Pregnancy and Delivery

© Copyright 2025– Jackie and Terry Mize

Printed in the United States of America. All rights reserved.

No portion of this book may be reproduced, stored in a retrieval system, or transmitted in any form or by any means—electronic, mechanical, photocopy, recording, scanning, or other—except for brief quotations in critical reviews or articles, without the prior written permission of the publisher. Unless otherwise identified, Scripture quotations are taken from the King James Version.

Scripture quotations marked AMPC are taken from the Amplified® Bible, Classic Edition, Copyright © 1954, 1958, 1962, 1964, 1965, 1987 by The Lockman Foundation. All rights reserved. Used by permission.

Scripture quotations marked NKJV are taken from the New King James Version. Copyright © 1982 by Thomas Nelson, Inc. Used by permission. All rights reserved.

Scripture quotations marked TLB are taken from The Living Bible; Tyndale House, 1997, © 1971 by Tyndale House Publishers, Inc. Used by permission. All rights reserved.

Scripture quotations marked CEV are taken from the Contemporary English Version Copyright © 1995 by the American Bible Society, New York, NY. All rights reserved.

Scripture quotations marked GNT are taken from the Good News Translation, Second Edition, Copyright 1992 by American Bible Society. Used by permission.

Scripture quotations marked CJB are taken from the Complete Jewish Bible, copyright © 1998 by David H. Stern. Published by Jewish New Testament Publications, Inc. www.messianicjewish.net/jntp. Distributed by Messianic Jewish Resources Int'l. www.messianicjewish.net. All rights reserved. Used by permission.

Scripture quotations marked YLT are taken from the 1898 Young's Literal Translation by Robert Young.

Published by Harrison House Publishers
Shippensburg, PA 17257

ISBN 13 TP: 978-1-6675-0928-0
ISBN 13 eBook: 978-1-6675-0929-7

For Worldwide Distribution, Printed in the U.S.A.

1 2 3 4 5 6 7 8 / 29 28 27 26 25

This Supernatural Childbirth Journal belongs to:

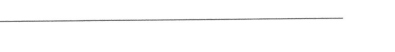

"Then God blessed them, and God said to them, 'Be fruitful and multiply...'"
(Genesis 1:28 NKJV).

DEDICATION TO JACKIE MIZE

In loving memory of Jackie Mize, who authored *Supernatural Childbirth* in 1993, sharing with women around the world the powerful truths of God's Word to help them conceive, enjoy healthy and happy pregnancies, and experience supernatural delivery.

The classic title from Harrison House recounts the personal testimony of how Jackie and her husband, Terry Mize, who had been told they could not have children, triumphed with four miracle children. What the couple learned and shared in *Supernatural Childbirth* went on to unlock powerful scriptural truths and dynamic faith principles for countless couples.

Today, Jackie would be delighted with this additional journal created as a companion to *Supernatural Childbirth* to walk hand-in-hand with women through their childbirth journey.

Jackie's legacy of courage and unwavering trust in God has left an indelible mark on lives across the globe. We honor her extraordinary contribution and pray that you, too, will experience the joys of pregnancy and delivery the supernatural way.

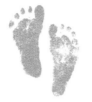

CONTENTS

A Personal Note from Terry Mize	1
How Do I Have Supernatural Childbirth?	3
Scriptures to Strengthen Your Faith	13
Discovering I'm Pregnant	17
Your Baby Is Known by God	18
A Prayer Confession for You	20
My Pregnancy Milestones	22
First Trimester Checklist	25
5 Weeks Pregnant	27
6 Weeks Pregnant	30
7 Weeks Pregnant	33
8 Weeks Pregnant	36
9 Weeks Pregnant	39
10 Weeks Pregnant	42
11 Weeks Pregnant	45

SUPERNATURAL CHILDBIRTH 40-WEEK PREGNANCY JOURNAL

12 Weeks Pregnant	48
Second Trimester Checklist	51
Nursery Planner	52
Nursery Essentials	53
13 Weeks Pregnant	58
14 Weeks Pregnant	61
15 Weeks Pregnant	64
16 Weeks Pregnant	67
17 Weeks Pregnant	70
18 Weeks Pregnant	73
19 Weeks Pregnant	76
20 Weeks Pregnant	79
20-Week Ultrasound	82
21 Weeks Pregnant	85
22 Weeks Pregnant	88
23 Weeks Pregnant	91
24 Weeks Pregnant	94
25 Weeks Pregnant	97
26 Weeks Pregnant	100
27 Weeks Pregnant	103
Third Trimester Checklist	106

Contents

28 Weeks Pregnant	107
29 Weeks Pregnant	110
30 Weeks Pregnant	113
31 Weeks Pregnant	116
32 Weeks Pregnant	119
33 Weeks Pregnant	122
34 Weeks Pregnant	125
35 Weeks Pregnant	128
36 Weeks Pregnant	131
37 Weeks Pregnant	134
38 Weeks Pregnant	137
39 Weeks Pregnant	140
40 Weeks Pregnant	143
Keeping Track of My Baby's Movements	147
Choosing My Baby's Name	152
A Letter to My Baby	153
My Prayer for My Baby's Future	154
My Baby Shower	155
Postpartum Checklist	156
My Birth Plan	157
Hospital Bag List	161

Arrival!	163
The Details	165
Home Sweet Home	166
Confessions and Prayers	168
Scriptures to Defeat Fear	170
Psalm 91 Confession	172
Psalm 103 Confession	174
During Pregnancy or Threatening Miscarriage	175
A Prayer for Baby Dedication	176

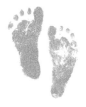

A PERSONAL NOTE FROM TERRY MIZE

To Jackie and me, the words "supernatural childbirth" weren't just a catchy phrase or a sermon title. These words to us meant Lynn, Paul, Lori, and Cristy. Supernatural childbirth to us meant faith in God's Word to bring about what man has declared impossible.

When Jackie and I met and began talking marriage, she said to me, "If we are going to get married, there is something about me you should know."

"*I can't have children!*" she said.

What a devastating statement! Women around the world have made the same declaration. My question to them now is the same question I posed to Jackie decades ago. "Oh, really? Who said? Who said you can't have children?" It makes a major difference in every area of your life—*who said*. I am always asking people that question, "Who said?"

Jackie answered me, "The doctors said."

"Oh, I see. Well, God said you can have babies," I told her. "Even though I thank God for doctors and hospitals, and medical science is always advancing, they are not our source, our final authority; God is, and God said you can have children."

"He did?"

"Sure. The Bible is full of Scriptures about children. He said He makes the barren woman to keep house and be a joyful mother of children. He said your children will be as olive plants and your wife as a fruitful vine. The Bible says there will be neither male nor female barren among God's people. We will have all the children we want."

And we did. We had four children—two boys and two girls. And we've taken them around the world with us, giving living bread to dying men, sharing the gospel with the world that cost the blood of Jesus.

Jackie's testimony of supernatural childbirth has gone literally around the world. In many nations where I go, people come up to me and say, "I've heard your late wife's teaching on supernatural childbirth." We have files of testimonies from women at home and abroad who have beautiful children because they applied these faith principles from God's Word. We strongly believe that any man, woman, boy, or girl can take God's Word and change his/her circumstances through faith and prayer.

Something that Jackie and I wanted people to understand is that to us, supernatural childbirth is being able to believe God to get pregnant, carry that baby to full term, and have a healthy mommy deliver a healthy baby. Many people think that supernatural childbirth only means having painless childbirth because that is what Jackie did with three of our four children, but we've never been dogmatic about that. Our point is having the baby and being healthy. The painless part and all the other extras we've had and believed for are available for you as you use your faith and "shoot for the stars; go for the best; aim high!" Those are faith principles. With God and faith, you can always go all out and aim high. The bottom line is this: the Bible says, "According to your faith." There isn't a right way and a wrong way in this book. There isn't "Jackie's way." It's according to your faith. We got what we used our faith for. We believe you will, too!

Terry L. Mize

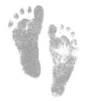

HOW DO I HAVE SUPERNATURAL CHILDBIRTH?

As you purpose in your heart to receive God's best in your pregnancy, you will discover that God will not disappoint. The Lord desires to bless and help you in every way! The key is knowing what God says and allowing His Word to override the things you were told or taught previously.

In her book *Supernatural Childbirth,* Jackie said:

> When Terry and I got married, May 10, 1969, we had so many things that looked like they were working against us. The doctor had told me for years that I'd never be able to have a baby at all—that I couldn't carry one. He said, "If by some slim chance you were ever going to get pregnant, you'd have to spend the whole nine months in bed. But even at that, I doubt that you could carry it." Well-meaning friends of the family and family members all said to Terry, "You know Jackie can't have children. It's really a shame, too, the way she loves babies and has always wanted to have a house full."
>
> We didn't know the word then like we do now, but Terry did know that God healed, and he knew some basics of the Bible from growing up in church. He knew we could pray and change things. Most of all, he knew God and knew that God's Word was always, and in every area, accurate. For all the years I've known him, his standard comment on any subject is "Who said?" It makes a big difference who said it. "What does God say? What does the Bible say?" So he told me, "I appreciate medical doctors and medical science.

They've come a long way, and I hope they go farther. But they are not our source, our answer, our final authority. God says we can have children. We'll have all the children we want."

We didn't know the details or the methods or exactly how to make it work in those early days, but we knew the will of God was to have children. It was His idea; He thought children up. He ordered them in the Garden of Eden. We knew that we could, that we would, have babies.

Begin to ask the same question. "What does God say? What does the Bible say about my pregnancy?" This question and the answers that follow will open the door for God to move. As God's Word becomes the focus, the expectations of pain, morning sickness, and long, agonizing deliveries are replaced by an expectation of God's blessing and supernatural power in the entire pregnancy and delivery.

Jackie explained:

> I want to clarify the difference between what I am calling "supernatural" childbirth and what everyone else calls "natural" childbirth. In natural childbirth classes, there are exercises. The woman is taught to center in on a focal point, to pant and breathe as directed, and the husband is taught to coach her through it, and so forth. This method does work to a degree, and praise God for it. Without it, many women would have had really bad experiences in giving birth. Natural childbirth is good, but God always has a better way of doing everything. Supernatural always exceeds natural in any area. And when we decide to do it His way, the results are amazing!
>
> When I refer to supernatural childbirth, I'm talking strictly about being able to conceive and to have babies with a pregnancy free from nausea, morning sickness, pain, moodiness, and depression, and without fear of any kind; then going through the entire labor without pain, and through the delivery without stitches and anesthetic. I'm talking about using the Word of God to overcome, change, and make things better.

How Do I Have Supernatural Childbirth?

You may be asking, "How do I do this? How do I have supernatural childbirth?" The following foundational truths will help you to receive God's supernatural help in your pregnancy.

1. You are redeemed from the curse and an heir of the blessing of God.
2. With God, all things are possible, including a supernatural childbirth.
3. God has given you His Word to produce the faith you need to receive His supernatural childbirth.

You Are Redeemed from "Sorrow" in Childbirth

God established childbirth in the very beginning as a part of His blessing. In His first words to man, He spoke about having a family, saying, *"Be fruitful, and multiply, and replenish the earth"* (Gen. 1:28). In God's original plan for pregnancy, we don't see any evidence of hard labors, pain, or sorrow. God made giving birth to children a part of the blessing!

So, when did "sorrow" become a part of childbirth? It entered because of the curse! When Adam and Eve sinned, their lives were completely changed. The blessing of God no longer governed them, but their lives became subject to the effects of the curse. In Genesis, the Lord explained how that would affect them, saying to Eve, *"I will greatly multiply thy sorrow and thy conception; in **sorrow** thou shalt bring forth children; and thy desire shall be to thy husband, and he shall rule over thee"* (Gen. 3:16).

But Jesus Christ redeemed you from the effects of the curse when He saved you. Galatians 3:13 declares, *"Christ hath redeemed us from the curse of the law, being made a curse for us: for it is written, Cursed is every one that hangeth on a tree."* The word *redeemed* includes the idea of "the payment of a price to recover one from the power of another." When Jesus was beaten with stripes on His back, He paid the price for our bodies to be redeemed from the curse.

*Surely he hath borne our griefs, and carried our **sorrows**: yet we did esteem him stricken, smitten of God, and afflicted. But he was wounded for our transgressions, he was bruised for our iniquities: the chastisement of our peace was upon him; and with his stripes we are healed* (Isaiah 53:4-5).

Every aspect of redemption must be received by faith. By faith, a person accepts the price Jesus paid to cleanse their sin. As a result of what they believe, they receive the new birth—they are born again! By faith, you believe that Jesus paid the price to free you from the effects of the curse, including sorrow in childbirth. As a result of your faith in what Jesus provided, the blessing of God governs the progress of your pregnancy.

That the blessing of Abraham might come on the Gentiles through Jesus Christ; that we might receive the promise of the Spirit through faith.

And if ye be Christ's, then are ye Abraham's seed, and heirs according to the promise (Galatians 3:14,29).

You are now an heir of the blessing of God. "*Surely blessing I will bless thee, and multiplying I will multiply thee*" (Heb. 6:14). You are a child of God with God's blessing as your inheritance. He wants you to trust in His blessing as you conceive. The Lord desires His blessing to cover every stage of your baby's development, and He wants you to rely on His blessing to flow as you give birth.

For Jackie Mize, the revelation of her redemption in Christ Jesus changed everything! She saw from God's Word that Jesus bore the sorrow and suffered every effect of the curse so that she could live free of it. Even though she had been told she would never be able to have a baby, Jackie realized she could trust God to help her conceive and carry her baby to term. She took her stand of faith that God's covenant set her apart from the pain, toil, and difficulties in pregnancy and childbirth, and God worked mightily on her behalf. To read Jackie's full testimony and teachings, read *Supernatural Childbirth: Experiencing the Promises of God Concerning Conception and Delivery.*

Embrace this truth today! You aren't subject to the curse but governed by the blessing of God. Believe that you will conceive and have a healthy, joyful pregnancy filled with peace and strength. Begin to expect the time of labor to be short and the delivery to be easy. You are an heir of the blessing of God through your relationship with Jesus Christ. Your pregnancy is subject to the blessing, and you are authorized to resist morning sickness and complications. You have the covenant right to believe that every aspect of your baby's development in the womb will progress as it should.

SUPERNATURAL CHILDBIRTH IS AVAILABLE TO YOU!

Terry and Jackie searched God's Word to locate the evidence they needed to build their faith in supernatural childbirth. Jackie said, "The reason it worked for us is we found it in God's Word and kept reading, studying, and talking it until it was a part of us."

A passage from the Book of Exodus caught their attention. The Hebrew women had their babies quickly and easily in comparison to the Egyptian women.

> *And the king of Egypt spake to the Hebrew midwives, of which the name of the one was Shiphrah, and the name of the other Puah:*
>
> *And he said, When ye do the office of a midwife to the Hebrew women, and see them upon the stools; if it be a son, then ye shall kill him: but if it be a daughter, then she shall live.*
>
> *But the midwives feared God, and did not as the king of Egypt commanded them, but saved the men children alive.*
>
> *And the king of Egypt called for the midwives, and said unto them, Why have ye done this thing, and have saved the men children alive?*

> *And the midwives said unto Pharaoh, Because the Hebrew women are not as the Egyptian women; **for they are lively**, and are delivered ere the midwives come in unto them* (Exodus 1:15-19).

That doesn't sound like sorrow in childbirth! The Hebrew women had easy labor and quick births, and so can you!

Let's compare the following translations of verse 19:

> *The midwives answered Pharaoh, Because the Hebrew women are not like the Egyptian women; they are vigorous and quickly delivered; their babies are born before the midwife comes to them* (Exodus 1:19 AMPC).

> *They give birth easily, and their babies are born before either of us gets there* (Exodus 1:19 GNT).

> *They go into labor and give birth before the midwife arrives* (Exodus 1:19 CJB).

You have a covenant with God, and the blessing belongs to you. The curse makes things hard, but the blessing of God makes your life great—including the birth of your baby!

In 1 Timothy 2:15, the Bible says, *"Notwithstanding she shall be saved in childbearing."* The word *saved* means kept safe and sound. Expect the blessing to prevail from the beginning of your pregnancy. Believe that you are saved from morning sickness, swollen ankles, mood swings, excruciating pain in labor, and complications in delivery.

GOD'S WORD WILL PRODUCE THE FAITH YOU NEED

Believing God for supernatural childbirth is not hard. Faith is a matter of planting God's Word in your heart until it produces a harvest of strong confidence. Through faith, you will receive the supernatural ability of God.

I can do all things through Christ which strengtheneth me (Philippians 4:13).

Jesus said unto him, If thou canst believe, all things are possible to him that believeth (Mark 9:23).

Then touched he their eyes, saying, According to your faith be it unto you (Matthew 9:29).

As you walk through each week of your pregnancy, deposit the Word of God consistently into your heart. Your heart will receive the seed of God's Word and produce a harvest of faith that God's blessing is protecting your baby and preparing your body for a supernatural birth.

With a heart full of God's Word, you are ready to declare God's Word over your body, your baby, and the delivery. Your words release the faith in your heart into the situation, activating the power of God. Romans 10:10 (AMPC) says, *"For with the heart a person believes (adheres to, trusts in, and relies on Christ) and so is justified (declared righteous, acceptable to God), and with the mouth he confesses (declares openly and speaks out freely his faith) and confirms [his] salvation."*

Jackie Mize emphasized the declaration of God's Word as an essential element of supernatural childbirth. She explained, "Confession is simply agreeing out loud with God, saying what God has already said. When we pray, we must pray the Word of God and pray in agreement with Him. We have God's Word for every area of our life; now it's up to us to make our own words agree with God's written Word."

The Bible says:

Death and life are in the power of the tongue: and they that love it shall eat the fruit thereof (Proverbs 18:21).

Thou art snared with the words of thy mouth, thou art taken with the words of thy mouth (Proverbs 6:2).

And this is the confidence that we have in him, that, if we ask any thing according to his will, he heareth us: and if we know that he hear us, whatsoever we ask, we know that we have the petitions that we desired of him (1 John 5:14-15).

For verily I say unto you, That whosoever shall say unto this mountain, Be thou removed, and be thou cast into the sea; and shall not doubt in his heart, but shall believe that those things which he saith shall come to pass; he shall have whatsoever he saith (Mark 11:23).

For out of the abundance of the heart the mouth speaketh (Matthew 12:34).

AGREE WITH GOD

In Amos 3:3, the Bible asks, *"Can two walk together, except they be agreed?"* When you find out what God has said about you and your baby, bring your thoughts, words, and actions into agreement with Him. Maintain the Word of God as the standard of what you expect to happen in this pregnancy and birth.

Every Word of God is full of power. Hebrews 4:12 (AMPC) says, *"For the Word that God speaks is alive and full of power [making it active, operative, energizing, and effective]."* As you speak God's Word, you release His life and power into your womb, your body, and the organs, ligaments, and tissues of your baby's body. Since the Word of God is voice-activated, you must speak the verses, not just read them. Speak to your baby in the womb and be as specific as you want. If you know of a problem in your family (heredity, sickness), you can address that. The important thing is that you are agreeing in faith with God and His Word. The concept of confession is not begging or pleading with God but thanking and agreeing with Him.

The following are some examples:

- Eyes: Vision, be perfect (Moses was 120 years old, and his eye wasn't dim).
- Ears: Hear perfectly.

- Skin: Complexion, be good.
- Teeth: Form perfectly. Be strong, not prone to cavities (Song of Solomon 4:2; 6:6).
- Bones: Be strong, healthy, straight, none broken (Ps. 34:20).
- Heart: Be strong, healthy, untroubled (John 14:1).
- Respiratory system: Be healthy and strong lungs and bronchial passages—no sinus problems, hay fever, or bronchitis.
- Blood: Be normal, and healthy. Maintain the proper blood sugar—no pollution in the blood (Ezek. 16:6).
- Digestive system: Function normally.
- Position of baby and cord: Baby, be head down and in perfect position at birth. Cord, be the perfect length and position, not around the baby's neck.
- Temperament: Be full of peace—a calm, sweet spirit and a tender heart (Isa. 54:13).
- Sleeping habits: Baby, you will sleep at night; you will get plenty of rest and let us rest.
- Baby's spirit: You will be tender toward God and the things of God, saved at an early age.

If parents or grandparents have a physical problem, don't confess that on your baby. Don't say, "It will have grandfather's teeth," or an aunt's complexion, or any family member's problems. But mirror God's Word to Him. Say to God and to you and to your mate and to your baby what God has already said, what God has already willed and written.

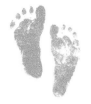

SCRIPTURES TO STRENGTHEN YOUR FAITH

These are the Scriptures used by Terry and Jackie Mize that established them in faith for supernatural childbirth. From the beginning, Jackie promised the Lord, "We will make our words agree with Your Word in every area—marriage, children, family, health, finances, ministry—and if we don't know what Your Word says on a given subject, we won't say anything until we look it up in the Bible, then we'll say what the Bible says."

> *This book of the law shall not depart out of thy mouth; but thou shalt meditate therein day and night, that thou mayest observe to do according to all that is written therein: for then thou shalt make thy way prosperous, and then thou shalt have good success* (Joshua 1:8).

> *Then said the Lord unto me, Thou hast well seen: for I will hasten my word to perform it* (Jeremiah 1:12).

> *I will worship toward thy holy temple, and praise thy name for thy lovingkindness and for thy truth: for thou hast magnified thy word above all thy name* (Psalm 138:2).

> *My son, attend to my words; incline thine ear unto my sayings. Let them not depart from thine eyes; keep them in the midst of thine heart. For they are life unto those that find them, and health to all their flesh* (Proverbs 4:20-22).

But my God shall supply all your need according to his riches in glory by Christ Jesus (Philippians 4:19).

For by him were all things created, that are in heaven, and that are in earth, visible and invisible, whether they be thrones, or dominions, or principalities, or powers: all things were created by him, and for him (Colossians 1:16).

The thief cometh not, but for to steal, and to kill, and to destroy: I am come that they might have life, and that they might have it more abundantly (John 10:10).

Thou art worthy, O Lord, to receive glory and honour and power: for thou hast created all things, and for thy pleasure they are and were created (Revelation 4:11).

Being confident of this very thing, that he which hath begun a good work in you will perform it until the day of Jesus Christ (Philippians 1:6).

Let us hold fast the profession of our faith without wavering; (for he is faithful that promised) (Hebrews 10:23).

Draw nigh to God, and he will draw nigh to you. Cleanse your hands, ye sinners; and purify your hearts, ye double minded (James 4:8).

Blessed is the man that walketh not in the counsel of the ungodly, nor standeth in the way of sinners, nor sitteth in the seat of the scornful. But his delight is in the law of the Lord; and in his law doth he meditate day and night. And he shall be like a tree planted by the rivers of water, that bringeth forth his fruit in his season; his leaf also shall not wither; and whatsoever he doeth shall prosper (Psalm 1:1-3).

And Jesus answered him, saying, It is written, That man shall not live by bread alone, but by every word of God (Luke 4:4).

Scriptures to Strengthen Your Faith

How God anointed Jesus of Nazareth with the Holy Ghost and with power: who went about doing good, and healing all that were oppressed of the devil; for God was with him (Acts 10:38).

For with the heart man believeth unto righteousness; and with the mouth confession is made unto salvation (Romans 10:10).

Nay, in all these things we are more than conquerors through him that loved us (Romans 8:37).

And be not conformed to this world: but be ye transformed by the renewing of your mind, that ye may prove what is that good, and acceptable, and perfect, will of God (Romans 12:2).

Who his own self bare our sins in his own body on the tree, that we, being dead to sins, should live unto righteousness: by whose stripes ye were healed (1 Peter 2:24).

Give, and it shall be given unto you; good measure, pressed down, and shaken together, and running over, shall men give into your bosom. For with the same measure that ye mete withal it shall be measured to you again (Luke 6:38).

Bring ye all the tithes into the storehouse, that there may be meat in mine house, and prove me now herewith, saith the Lord of hosts, if I will not open you the windows of heaven, and pour you out a blessing, that there shall not be room enough to receive it. And I will rebuke the devourer for your sakes, and he shall not destroy the fruits of your ground; neither shall your vine cast her fruit before the time in the field, saith the Lord of hosts (Malachi 3:10-11).

Beloved, I wish above all things that thou mayest prosper and be in health, even as thy soul prospereth (3 John 2).

Surely he hath borne our griefs, and carried our sorrows: yet we did esteem him stricken, smitten of God, and afflicted. But he was wounded for our transgressions, he was bruised for our iniquities: the chastisement of our peace was upon him; and with his stripes we are healed (Isaiah 53:4-5).

And all thy children shall be taught of the Lord; and great shall be the peace of thy children. In righteousness shalt thou be established: thou shalt be far from oppression; for thou shalt not fear: and from terror; for it shall not come near thee. Behold, they shall surely gather together, but not by me: whosoever shall gather together against thee shall fall for thy sake (Isaiah 54:13-15).

No weapon that is formed against thee shall prosper; and every tongue that shall rise against thee in judgment thou shalt condemn. This is the heritage of the servants of the Lord, and their righteousness is of me, saith the Lord (Isaiah 54:17).

Use the following verses from Galatians to negate the curses of the Law found especially in Deuteronomy chapter 28.

Christ hath redeemed us from the curse of the law, being made a curse for us: for it is written, Cursed is every one that hangeth on a tree: that the blessing of Abraham might come on the Gentiles through Jesus Christ; that we might receive the promise of the Spirit through faith. …And if ye be Christ's, then are ye Abraham's seed, and heirs according to the promise (Galatians 3:13-14,29).

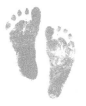

DISCOVERING I'M PREGNANT

Date I found out: _____

Symptoms:

_____
_____
_____
_____

Who I first told about my pregnancy and how they reacted

_____
_____
_____
_____

Things God put in my heart to pray about my baby's future

_____
_____
_____
_____

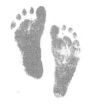

YOUR BABY IS KNOWN BY GOD

Before I formed thee in the belly I knew thee; and before thou camest forth out of the womb I sanctified thee, and I ordained thee a prophet unto the nations (Jeremiah 1:5).

In the Bible, we find that babies, even in the womb (uterus), were real and alive and known to God. Luke 1:41 says of John the Baptist, "*And it came to pass, that, when Elisabeth heard the salutation of Mary, the babe leaped in her womb; and Elisabeth was filled with the Holy Ghost.*"

In Genesis 25:23, God told Rebekah of her boys in her womb that, "*Two nations are in thy womb, and two manner of people shall be separated from thy bowels; and the one people shall be stronger than the other people; and the elder shall serve the younger.*"

God didn't just see "fetuses." He saw men and the nations they would become. For example, in Judges 13:5-7, God said that Samson was a Nazirite from the womb to the day of his death.

Here are some additional verses that reveal God's intimacy with babies in the womb.

For thou hast possessed my reins: thou hast covered me in my mother's womb (Psalm 139:13).

Thus saith the Lord that made thee, and formed thee from the womb, which will help thee; Fear not, O Jacob, my servant; and thou, Jesurun, whom I have chosen (Isaiah 44:2).

Your Baby Is Known by God

But when it pleased God, who separated me from my mother's womb, and called me by his grace (Galatians 1:15).

Your baby has a destiny and purpose in God. Open your heart to pray in line with God's plan for your baby. Celebrate the life of God in your womb and the bright, blessed future your child has in store.

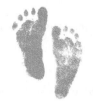

A PRAYER CONFESSION FOR YOU

Thank You, Father, for this child. I can say with Hannah, "For this child I prayed and the Lord hath given me my petition which I asked of him."

Thank You, Lord, for a wonderful pregnancy, an enjoyable pregnancy. Thank You that I am in control over my body and the Word has preeminence in my life. I will not be subject to my emotions, but they are subject to Your Word. I'll not have morning sickness. You said You bless my bread and water and take sickness out of my midst. Not only will I enjoy this pregnancy, but my family will, as well. It will be a good time, a pleasant time. I'll rest well and sleep well. You said You give Your beloved sleep. I'll watch what I eat and not gain too much weight. The children of Israel walked forty years in the wilderness and their feet didn't swell; my feet will not swell in Jesus' name. Thank You for what Your Word calls blessings of the breasts and of the womb (Gen. 49:25). I'll not have sore or cracked nipples and breasts.

I will feel and be feminine. I radiate life. I glow and am attractive during this pregnancy. My husband and children will enjoy being with me, and I will enjoy being with them. I'll be amorous and loving toward my husband. Your Word says that he is always ravished with my love and my breasts satisfy him at all times. He has no need of spoil during this time and he drinks waters out of his own well, and he rejoices with the wife of his youth, the wife of his covenant—me! We will continue to have a good and blessed sex life during this pregnancy!

A Prayer Confession for You

This pregnancy will be full duration, full term. I'm a tither, and my vine won't cast its fruit before its time in the field. You said I would not cast my young or miscarry and the number of my days You would fulfill. Thank You that You bless the fruit of my womb. My baby is covered in my womb as David declared. You said numerous times in the Bible that You formed and fashioned our baby in the womb and at the right time You will separate my baby from my womb and carry it gently from my womb.

Father, I declare over this precious one, as I do over all my family, that we are healed by the stripes of Jesus. No sickness, no plague, no evil can come upon us. Your angels have charge over us and keep us in all our ways and lift us up lest we dash our foot against a stone. Just like all the ladies of faith in the Bible, I will give birth to a healthy, whole baby, a child whose heart is toward God and Your promise. And Your command is that if we train this child up in the way he/she should go, he/she won't depart from it when he/she is old. Our baby will honor his/her father and mother and obey; therefore, it will be well (not sick) with our child, and he/she will live long on the earth.

Father, I speak to my body and to my baby—to every part, every organ, every system to function properly and perfectly, fully developed as You intended from the beginning. I declare health, wholeness, soundness, spirit, soul, and body from the top of the head to the bottom of the feet.

We pray for the medical professionals we are involved with, that they have the mind of Christ and wisdom of God concerning our family and this baby. The eyes of their understanding be opened that You, Father, lead and guide them how to care for me/my wife by Your Spirit. I say we have favor with them, that they are cooperative with us and what we are doing, that all is well and peaceful and under control in Jesus' name.

Thank You, Father, for this time for our family and time to spend with You. Thank You for fulfilling Your promise in Your Word. In Jesus' name. Amen (1 Sam. 1:27; Ex. 23:25; Ps. 127:2; Deut. 8:4; Gen. 49:25; Prov. 5:19; Prov. 5:15; Mal. 3:11; Ex. 23:26; Deut. 7:13; Ps. 139:13; Isa. 44:2; Gal. 1:15; Jer. 1:5; Ps. 71:6; Ps. 22:9-10; 1 Peter 2:24; Ps. 91:10-12; Prov. 22:6; Eph. 6:2-3; 3 John 2; Ezek. 16:6; Isa. 54:13; Eph. 1:17-18; Prov. 3:3-4).

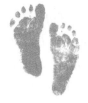

MY PREGNANCY MILESTONES

As you share your milestone moments in the lines below, don't forget to include the dates!

I'm pregnant! Date I found out: _____

Today, I heard the heartbeat: _____

What I want to remember most about how I felt in that moment:

_____

_____

_____

_____

_____

We know our baby's gender! I'm having a _____

I felt the baby move today! What I want to remember most about this miraculous moment and tell my child about someday!

_____

_____

_____

_____

_____

My Pregnancy Milestones

- Date of my first ultrasound: _____
- I'm saving my first ultrasound picture below. Here are my first thoughts when I *saw* my baby!

Attach ultrasound picture here.

_____
_____
_____
_____
_____
_____
_____
_____

- How we've celebrated the news of our pregnancy!

Attach picture here.

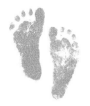

FIRST TRIMESTER CHECKLIST

Let's get started!

- My doctor's name is _____
- My due date is _____
- Start a prenatal vitamin
- Consider foods to avoid
- Plan your pregnancy announcement
- Begin taking baby "bump" photos

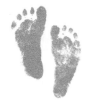

MY PRAYER FOCUS AND FAITH CONFESSION

I will worship toward thy holy temple, and praise thy name for thy lovingkindness and for thy truth: for thou hast magnified thy word above all thy name (Psalm 138:2).

Father, in Jesus' name, I enter Your presence with thanksgiving and praise. I celebrate the plan You have for my baby and the blessing of a supernatural pregnancy. I honor Your Word as the final authority in my life. Your Word governs my pregnancy and has pre-eminence in my life! I agree with Your Word that I am redeemed from the curse because Jesus was cursed in my place. I am not subject to my emotions, but they are subject to Your Word. I'll not have morning sickness because You said You bless my bread and water and take sickness out of my midst. I am an heir of the blessing, and Your blessing is the supernatural force governing my body, the baby in my womb, and even my delivery. Thank You, God, for Your Word!

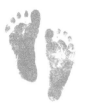

5 WEEKS PREGNANT

- Today's date: _____

- My current weight: _____

- My belly measurement: _____

- My scripture focus:

_____
_____
_____
_____
_____
_____
_____
_____
_____
_____
_____

SUPERNATURAL CHILDBIRTH 40-WEEK PREGNANCY JOURNAL

- What I'm thinking and feeling most at this milestone of my pregnancy!

_____
_____
_____
_____
_____
_____
_____
_____

Attach photo or memento here

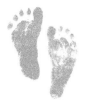

MY PRAYER FOCUS AND FAITH CONFESSION

*(As it is written, I have made thee a father of many nations,) before him whom he believed, even God, who quickeneth the dead, and **calleth those things which be not as though they were*** (Romans 4:17).

Lord, I will follow the example You have given me in Romans 4:17. I will hold my mouth in line with Your Word and call things as though they were. I declare that my child is fearfully and wonderfully made, perfectly formed, and healthy. I call my body strong. I am free from morning sickness because I am redeemed from the curse. I will enjoy this pregnancy and so will my family because it will be a good, pleasant time. Father, I ask You to give me the tongue of the learned (Isa. 50:4) and fill my mouth with the things I need to say.

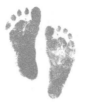

6 WEEKS PREGNANT

- Today's date: _____

- My current weight: _____

- My belly measurement: _____

- My scripture focus:

_____

_____

_____

_____

_____

_____

_____

_____

_____

6 Weeks Pregnant

- What I'm thinking and feeling most at this milestone of my pregnancy!

_____
_____
_____
_____
_____
_____
_____
_____
_____

Attach photo or memento here

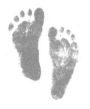

MY PRAYER FOCUS AND FAITH CONFESSION

*For the Word that God speaks is alive and full of power [making it **active, operative, energizing, and effective**]* (Hebrews 4:12 AMPC).

Father, I thank You for providing Your Word so that I can establish Your will in my pregnancy. Your Word is active in my body, strengthening my womb. I speak Your Word to operate in my bloodstream and carry all that my baby needs to be strong and healthy. I declare Your Word, saying, "I am strong in the Lord and in the power of Your might. I will rest well because the Lord gives His beloved sleep" (Ps. 127:2). This pregnancy will be to full term because I am a tither, and my vine won't cast its fruit before its time in the field (Mal. 3:11). You said I would not cast my young or miscarry and the number of my days You would fulfill (Ex. 23:26). Lord, Your Word energizes my spirit. I ask You to teach me how to put your Word to work to set the course of my pregnancy and delivery.

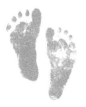

7 WEEKS PREGNANT

- Today's date: _____

- My current weight: _____

- My belly measurement: _____

- My scripture focus:

_____
_____
_____
_____
_____
_____
_____
_____
_____
_____

Supernatural Childbirth 40-Week Pregnancy Journal

- What I'm thinking and feeling most at this milestone of my pregnancy!

_____
_____
_____
_____
_____
_____
_____
_____

Attach photo or memento here

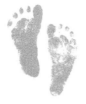

MY PRAYER FOCUS AND FAITH CONFESSION

By faith we understand that the worlds [during the successive ages] **were framed (fashioned, put in order, and equipped for their intended purpose)** *by the word of God, so that what we see was not made out of things which are visible* (Hebrews 11:3 AMPC).

Father, You used Your Word to create all things and direct the universe to operate the way You want it to work. You have given me Your Word to frame my world, put it in the correct order, and equip my life for Your purpose. In the name of Jesus, I declare my womb is blessed, and I call my body strong. I speak to the child in my womb, saying, "God perfects that which concerns you. Your heart is strong! Your brain is healthy and blessed. Your joints are limber, and every system forms with the perfection of God. You are healed by the stripes of Jesus, and no sickness, disease, or plague can come near you." Father, I frame my pregnancy and the delivery of my child with Your promise that You will strengthen me. You will help me. You will uphold me with the right hand of Your righteousness (Isa. 41:10).

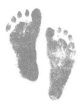

8 WEEKS PREGNANT

- Today's date: _____

- My current weight: _____

- My belly measurement: _____

- My scripture focus:

_____
_____
_____
_____
_____
_____
_____
_____
_____
_____

8 Weeks Pregnant

- What I'm thinking and feeling most at this milestone of my pregnancy!

_____
_____
_____
_____
_____
_____
_____
_____
_____

Attach photo or memento here

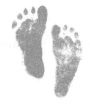

MY PRAYER FOCUS AND FAITH CONFESSION

And he will love thee, and bless thee, and multiply thee: he will also bless the fruit of thy womb, and the fruit of thy land, thy corn, and thy wine, and thine oil, the increase of thy kine, and the flocks of thy sheep, in the land which he sware unto thy fathers to give thee (Deuteronomy 7:13).

Heavenly Father, I am so grateful for the love You have for me and my baby. Your blessing on our lives is so amazing. As I lay my hands on my tummy, I call my baby blessed. Every cell in my child's body is under the power of Your blessing. As my baby forms, it forms perfectly healthy and strong. My body is submitted to the force of the blessing. I resist weakness and morning sickness in the name of Jesus. I radiate the life of God! Lord, You preserved the children of Israel in the wilderness so that their feet did not swell. You are no respecter of persons, so I declare my feet will not swell. I resist any negative mood swings or problems with blood pressure or blood sugar in the name of Jesus. Your peace governs my pregnancy and **supernatural childbirth**. *I rejoice in Your redemption in Jesus' name.*

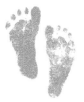

9 WEEKS PREGNANT

- Today's date: _____

- My current weight: _____

- My belly measurement: _____

- My scripture focus:

_____
_____
_____
_____
_____
_____
_____
_____
_____
_____
_____

Supernatural Childbirth 40-Week Pregnancy Journal

- What I'm thinking and feeling most at this milestone of my pregnancy!

_____
_____
_____
_____
_____
_____
_____
_____
_____

Attach photo or memento here

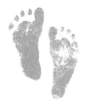

MY PRAYER FOCUS AND FAITH CONFESSION

Lo, children are an heritage of the Lord: and the fruit of the womb is his reward (Psalm 127:3).

In the name of Jesus, I thank You for this life in my womb. Heavenly Father, I recognize You as the Life Giver and Creator. I seek You for the wisdom to lead my child in Your paths. I declare that I will give birth to a healthy child whose heart is turned toward You and Your Word. I will train up this child in the way that he/she should go and he/she won't depart from Your ways. My child will honor his/her father and mother and obey us. Therefore, it will be well with my child and he/she will live long on the earth (Eph. 6:2-3). Let Your wisdom overflow in me so I can help my child know Your greatness, salvation, and love for us. Cultivate in me the patience and understanding to guide, train, and prepare my child for the great things You have planned. Lord, let Your will be done in my child's life.

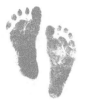

10 WEEKS PREGNANT

- Today's date: _____

- My current weight: _____

- My belly measurement: _____

- My scripture focus:

_____
_____
_____
_____
_____
_____
_____
_____
_____
_____

10 Weeks Pregnant

- What I'm thinking and feeling most at this milestone of my pregnancy!

_____
_____
_____
_____
_____
_____
_____
_____
_____

Attach photo or memento here

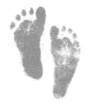

MY PRAYER FOCUS AND FAITH CONFESSION

My son, attend to my words; incline thine ear unto my sayings. Let them not depart from thine eyes; keep them in the midst of thine heart. For they are life unto those that find them, and health to all their flesh (Proverbs 4:20-22).

Father, in the name of Jesus, I give my attention to Your Word today. I incline my ear to hear and purposefully put Your Word in my eyes. I maintain the fullness of my heart with Your promises because Your Word is life to my baby and health to the bones, organs, muscles, and tissue of my child. I speak to my baby right now and command that every organ and system in your body will function properly and perfectly. Be fully developed and work to God's perfect standard. I declare health, wholeness, and soundness in every area. Eyes, be perfectly formed. Ears, you will hear perfectly. Bones, be strong and healthy in the name of Jesus. Thank You, Lord, for giving me the ability to use Your words and the authority in Jesus' name.

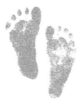

11 WEEKS PREGNANT

- Today's date: _____

- My current weight: _____

- My belly measurement: _____

- My scripture focus:

_____
_____
_____
_____
_____
_____
_____
_____
_____
_____
_____
_____

SUPERNATURAL CHILDBIRTH 40-WEEK PREGNANCY JOURNAL

- What I'm thinking and feeling most at this milestone of my pregnancy!

_____
_____
_____
_____
_____
_____
_____
_____
_____

Attach photo or memento here

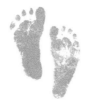

MY PRAYER FOCUS AND FAITH CONFESSION

But he was wounded for our transgressions, he was bruised for our iniquities: the chastisement of our peace was upon him; and with his stripes we are healed (Isaiah 53:5).

In the name of Jesus, I rejoice in Your redemption. Jesus took the stripes on His back to purchase my healing and even the health of my child. He was wounded and bruised so that I could be healed and whole. Thank You for this covenant supply that frees me from suffering in childbirth. I release my faith in this provision, declaring, "I receive the price Jesus paid when He was wounded for my transgressions. **Supernatural childbirth** *is my heritage because the punishment necessary to obtain my well-being was upon Jesus." I pray and confess that my body and my baby will cooperate with perfect, supernatural delivery, and there will be no problems of any kind. According to Psalm 103, the Lord redeems my life from destruction. He heals all my diseases and crowns me and my child with His loving-kindness and tender mercies. Thank You, Father, for Your blessing over my pregnancy. I believe Your highest and best is at work in my life.*

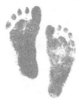

12 WEEKS PREGNANT

- Today's date: _____

- My current weight: _____

- My belly measurement: _____

- My scripture focus:
_____
_____
_____
_____
_____
_____
_____
_____
_____
_____

12 Weeks Pregnant

- What I'm thinking and feeling most at this milestone of my pregnancy!

_____
_____
_____
_____
_____
_____
_____
_____
_____

Attach photo or memento here

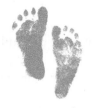

MY PRAYER FOCUS AND FAITH CONFESSION

That it might be fulfilled which was spoken by Esaias the prophet, saying, Himself took our infirmities, and bare our sicknesses (Matthew 8:17).

I worship You, Lord, for taking sickness and disease out of my life. You are the Lord who heals me (Ex. 15:26). I declare Your health and life are flowing freely through my body into the baby in my womb. We are governed by Matthew 8:17 and established in health. I am free from moodiness, depression, and morning sickness because Jesus took my infirmities. My pregnancy is blessed by God, full of health, peace, and joy! I confess my body will cooperate with the blessing of God and resist all symptoms associated with the curse, sickness, or disease. My body and my baby will experience a perfect and **supernatural childbirth** with a quick, easy, and painless delivery. Since Jesus bore our sickness, my baby and I are well, whole, and thriving. In Jesus' name, my child is strong and developing perfectly and on track.

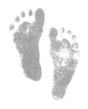

SECOND TRIMESTER CHECKLIST

Halfway there!

- Plan your nursery
- Plan maternity leave
- Schedule second trimester prenatal visits and tests
- Choose a pediatrician
- Consider childcare options
- Moisturize your tummy
- Set up a baby registry for baby shower
- Purchase maternity clothes

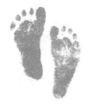

NURSERY PLANNER

Theme Ideas	
Color Scheme Ideas	
Furniture Pieces	

Nursery Checklist

- Decide on theme and color scheme
- Purchase or register decor in baby registry
- Purchase or register nursery furniture
- Arrange and organize
- Baby-proof the nursery

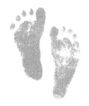

NURSERY ESSENTIALS

BEDTIME

- ☐ Crib
- ☐ Crib mattress
- ☐ Crib liner
- ☐ Mattress protectors
- ☐ Bed sheets
- ☐ Bassinet
- ☐ Baby monitor
- ☐ White-noise machine

BREAST FEEDING

- ☐ Nursing pillow
- ☐ Nursing bras
- ☐ Breast pads
- ☐ Nursing covers
- ☐ Nipple cream
- ☐ Breast pump
- ☐ Burp cloths
- ☐ Milk storage containers

Bathing

- ☐ Baby tub
- ☐ Baby bath set
- ☐ Hooded towels
- ☐ Baby shampoo
- ☐ Baby lotion
- ☐ Baby oil
- ☐ Baby body wash
- ☐ Non-slip bathmat
- ☐ Bath thermometer
- ☐ Soft sponge
- ☐ Bath toys
- ☐ Bath toy storage
- ☐ Nail clippers

Furniture

- ☐ Changing table
- ☐ Baby hangers
- ☐ Dresser
- ☐ Rocking chair
- ☐ Baby seat
- ☐ Baby bouncer
- ☐ Hamper
- ☐ Travel crib
- ☐ Blackout curtains

Nursery Essentials

CHANGING

- ☐ Changing mat
- ☐ Diapers
- ☐ Baby wipes
- ☐ Night-light
- ☐ Diaper rash cream
- ☐ Sealable bin
- ☐ Disposable bin bags
- ☐ Pee-pee tepee (boys)

FEEDING

- ☐ Bottles
- ☐ Bottle nipples
- ☐ Baby formula
- ☐ Bottle brush
- ☐ Bottle warmer
- ☐ Sterilizer kit
- ☐ Mild dish soap
- ☐ Bibs
- ☐ Burp cloths
- ☐ Food storage containers
- ☐ Food processor
- ☐ Highchair
- ☐ Baby bowls/plates/utensils
- ☐ Baby cups
- ☐ Drying rack

Clothing

- ☐ Onesies
- ☐ T-shirts
- ☐ Pants/leggings
- ☐ Gowns/sleepers
- ☐ Hats
- ☐ Socks
- ☐ Jackets
- ☐ Dressy clothes

Health Items

- ☐ Baby thermometer
- ☐ Humidifier
- ☐ Sunscreen
- ☐ Medicine spoon/syringe
- ☐ Nasal aspirator
- ☐ First aid kit

Safety Items

- ☐ Outlet covers
- ☐ TV furniture wall straps
- ☐ Baby gate
- ☐ Drawer/cabinet locks
- ☐ Door handle locks
- ☐ Window locks
- ☐ Backseat car mirror
- ☐ Car window shade

Nursery Essentials

Toys

- ☐ Activity mat
- ☐ Rattle
- ☐ Cuddle toys
- ☐ Teething toys
- ☐ Sensory toys
- ☐ Musical toys
- ☐ Pacifier toys
- ☐ Stroller toys
- ☐ Crib mobile

Additional Items

- ☐ Car seat
- ☐ Playpen
- ☐ Soft toy/comforter
- ☐ Diaper bag
- ☐ Stroller
- ☐ Baby carrier
- ☐ Thermal bottle carrier

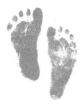

13 WEEKS PREGNANT

- Today's date: _____

- My current weight: _____

- My belly measurement: _____

- My scripture focus:

_____
_____
_____
_____
_____
_____
_____
_____
_____
_____

13 Weeks Pregnant

- What I'm thinking and feeling most at this milestone of my pregnancy!

_____
_____
_____
_____
_____
_____
_____
_____
_____

Attach photo or memento here

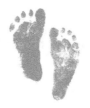

MY PRAYER FOCUS AND FAITH CONFESSION

For You formed my inward parts; You covered me in my mother's womb (Psalm 139:13 NKJV).

Father, I worship You for Your handiwork in my womb. You are personally guiding and perfecting the growth and development of every organ in my baby's body. I worship You, Lord, for my baby is fearfully and wonderfully made. I speak health and life to my baby. I speak to the formation of every cell, tissue, and organ and I command you to thrive with the life of God. I declare the blessing of God over the organs of my baby. Heart, be blessed. Lungs, be strong. Brain, form perfectly. Digestive system, endocrine system, blood steam, be blessed and thrive with the life and blessing of the Lord, in the name of Jesus! Lord, according to Psalm 91, because I set my love on You, You will deliver me. You will set me on high because I have known Your name. If I call on You, You will answer me. You will be with me in trouble, deliver me, and honor me! Thank You for being my ever-present Help.

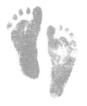

14 WEEKS PREGNANT

- Today's date: _____
- My current weight: _____
- My belly measurement: _____
- My scripture focus:

_____
_____
_____
_____
_____
_____
_____
_____
_____
_____

- What I'm thinking and feeling most at this milestone of my pregnancy!

_____
_____
_____
_____
_____
_____
_____
_____
_____

Attach photo or memento here

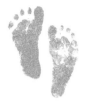

MY PRAYER FOCUS AND FAITH CONFESSION

I will praise You, for I am fearfully and wonderfully made; marvelous are Your works, and that my soul knows very well (Psalm 139:14 NKJV).

*I lift up my voice to praise You, Lord. You are the Life-Giver, and marvelous are Your works. You have formed this beautiful child in my womb and blessed me to be a joyful mother of children (Ps. 113:9). Thank You, Father! You have equipped me with exceeding great and precious promises that include **supernatural childbirth**. In the name of Jesus, I strengthen myself in Your Word. I confess, "I am redeemed from the curse because Jesus was cursed for me. I am free from morning sickness. I am redeemed from swollen ankles and mood swings." Lord, You have designed me to live under the blessing of health and strength. I declare, "You are my strength and my shield. I resist every physical symptom, emotional heaviness, worry, or anxiety because the kingdom of heaven is righteousness, peace, and joy in the Holy Ghost" (Rom. 14:17). I praise You for redeeming me from the curse and making me an heir of the blessing!*

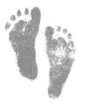

15 WEEKS PREGNANT

- Today's date: _____

- My current weight: _____

- My belly measurement: _____

- My scripture focus:

_____
_____
_____
_____
_____
_____
_____
_____
_____
_____

15 Weeks Pregnant

- What I'm thinking and feeling most at this milestone of my pregnancy!

_____
_____
_____
_____
_____
_____
_____
_____

Attach photo or memento here

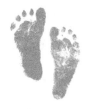

MY PRAYER FOCUS AND FAITH CONFESSION

[Most] blessed is the man who believes in, trusts in, and relies on the Lord, and whose hope and confidence the Lord is. For he shall be like a tree planted by the waters that spreads out its roots by the river; and it shall not see and fear when heat comes; but its leaf shall be green. It shall not be anxious and full of care in the year of drought, nor shall it cease yielding fruit (Jeremiah 17:7-8 AMPC).

Heavenly Father, I trust in You with all my heart. I depend on You and Your Word to direct this supernatural pregnancy. I am confident that You have freed me from the curse. I am not obligated to suffer long, difficult, painful childbirth. In the name of Jesus, I don't have to endure months of fatigue during pregnancy or postpartum depression after the birth of my child. According to Colossians 1:13, I have been delivered from the power of darkness, and I have been translated (completely relocated) into the kingdom of God's dear Son. I expect to be energetic and well-rested throughout each trimester. My blood sugar levels will remain normal, and I will be active until I am ready to deliver. In the name of Jesus, I command my body to submit to the Word of God and cooperate with the blessing. I declare that I rest well and sleep well. Praise You, Lord, for giving me health and causing me to thrive!

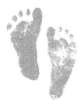

16 WEEKS PREGNANT

- Today's date: _____

- My current weight: _____

- My belly measurement: _____

- My scripture focus:

_____
_____
_____
_____
_____
_____
_____
_____
_____
_____

SUPERNATURAL CHILDBIRTH 40-WEEK PREGNANCY JOURNAL

- What I'm thinking and feeling most at this milestone of my pregnancy!

_____
_____
_____
_____
_____
_____
_____
_____

Attach photo or memento here

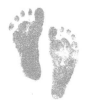

MY PRAYER FOCUS AND FAITH CONFESSION

In righteousness shalt thou be established: thou shalt be far from oppression; for thou shalt not fear: and from terror; for it shall not come near thee (Isaiah 54:14).

Father, I come to You today in the name of Jesus. Because Jesus was made to be sin for me, I have been made the righteousness of God in Him. Jesus has made me righteous, and I am established in Him by faith. I exercise my authority in Jesus' name to resist oppression and fear. I set myself against any fear or dread of experiencing pain in labor. According to Isaiah 53:4 (YLT), "Surely our sicknesses he hath borne, and our pains—he hath carried them." Since Jesus bore my pains, I expect to have a painless pregnancy and delivery. As my body changes and my baby grows, I don't have to suffer pain. I declare that I won't suffer labor pains when my muscles contract in the delivery of my baby. I cast down every imagination of suffering and difficulty in childbirth that is based on movies I've seen or stories I've heard. God has not given me a spirit of fear, but of power, and of love, and of a sound mind (2 Tim. 1:7). I have God's perfect love, and that perfect love casts out fear.

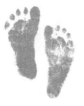

17 WEEKS PREGNANT

- Today's date: _____

- My current weight: _____

- My belly measurement: _____

- My scripture focus:

_____
_____
_____
_____
_____
_____
_____
_____
_____
_____

17 Weeks Pregnant

- What I'm thinking and feeling most at this milestone of my pregnancy!

_____
_____
_____
_____
_____
_____
_____
_____
_____

Attach photo or memento here

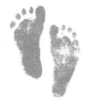

MY PRAYER FOCUS AND FAITH CONFESSION

For out of the abundance of the heart the mouth speaketh. A good man out of the good treasure of the heart bringeth forth good things (Matthew 12:34–35).

Lord, I commit to keep my words in line with Yours. Help me to speak accurately about my birth and pregnancy when I share things with others or discuss things with my doctor. I will not use my words to rehearse horror stories of long, painful labors. I will not tell stories or have discussions about conditions or complications that other people have suffered in childbirth. According to James 3:2, I can bridle my body by using my words correctly, so teach me to use words that direct my pregnancy in the path of the blessing. I declare that my pregnancy is submitted to the authority of God's Word. Your Word says that I am saved in childbirth and redeemed from the curse. Since pain in childbirth came as a result of the curse, I resist it with the shield of faith. In the name of Jesus, I pray Psalm 141:3, "Set a watch, O Lord, before my mouth; keep the door of my lips." I purpose to fill my heart with daily deposits of Your Word, specific verses that produce faith in Your redemption and supernatural provision.

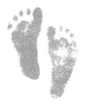

18 WEEKS PREGNANT

- Today's date: _____

- My current weight: _____

- My belly measurement: _____

- My scripture focus:

_____
_____
_____
_____
_____
_____
_____
_____
_____
_____

Supernatural Childbirth 40-Week Pregnancy Journal

- What I'm thinking and feeling most at this milestone of my pregnancy!

_____
_____
_____
_____
_____
_____
_____
_____
_____

Attach photo or memento here

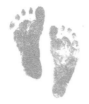

MY PRAYER FOCUS AND FAITH CONFESSION

Let the words of my mouth, and the meditation of my heart, be acceptable in thy sight, O Lord, my strength, and my redeemer (Psalm 19:14).

*Father, as I prepare for supernatural childbirth, I commit my ways to You. I choose to present myself to You as a living sacrifice. I act on Your Word in Romans 12:2, and I renew my mind so that I may prove what Your good, acceptable, and perfect will is. I choose thoughts from Your list in Philippians 4:8—whatsoever things are true, honest, just, pure, lovely, whatsoever things are of good report; if there be any virtue, and if there be any praise, I will think on these things! That means when I think about the delivery of my baby, I will expect to deliver like the Hebrew women described in Exodus 1:19, "the Hebrew women are not as the Egyptian women; for they are lively, and are delivered ere the midwives come in unto them." I expect Your favor to surround me during this entire pregnancy and even in the delivery room. I anticipate a **supernatural childbirth**, in Jesus' name!*

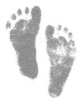

19 WEEKS PREGNANT

- Today's date: _____

- My current weight: _____

- My belly measurement: _____

- My scripture focus:

_____
_____
_____
_____
_____
_____
_____
_____
_____
_____

19 Weeks Pregnant

- What I'm thinking and feeling most at this milestone of my pregnancy!

_____
_____
_____
_____
_____
_____
_____
_____
_____

Attach photo or memento here

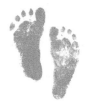

MY PRAYER FOCUS AND FAITH CONFESSION

The Lord will perfect that which concerneth me: thy mercy, O Lord, endureth for ever (Psalm 138:8).

Heavenly Father, You are so faithful in preparing the way for me and providing all of the wisdom and strength that I may need. You perfect the things concerning me, my pregnancy and delivery. I trust You to lead me in every decision. Concerning the decisions that need to be made and the supplies that need to be gathered, I refuse to allow them to be a burden. I guard my peace and joy and depend on Your wisdom to help me. So, I declare, "In Jesus' name, I refuse to be overwhelmed or burdened with the preparations that I need to make. I cast my cares on the Lord because He cares for me." I thank You because You give me victory through my Lord Jesus Christ (1 Cor. 15:58), and You always cause me to triumph in Christ (2 Cor. 2:14). In every situation, You have the answers I need. Thank You, Lord!

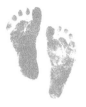

20 WEEKS PREGNANT

- Today's date: _____

- My current weight: _____

- My belly measurement: _____

- My scripture focus:

_____

_____

_____

_____

_____

_____

_____

_____

_____

_____

SUPERNATURAL CHILDBIRTH 40-WEEK PREGNANCY JOURNAL

- What I'm thinking and feeling most at this milestone of my pregnancy!

_____
_____
_____
_____
_____
_____
_____
_____
_____

Attach photo or memento here

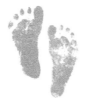

MY PRAYER FOCUS AND FAITH CONFESSION

And this is the confidence that we have in him, that, if we ask any thing according to his will, he heareth us (1 John 5:14).

*What a privilege it is to have You as my Heavenly Father, my God. Instead of being anxious about anything, I can make my petition known to You. I can come confidently to Your throne and receive help in my time of need. You instruct me to ask in faith and receive from You. I receive Your supernatural help in this pregnancy. I ask You to strengthen the baby in my womb. Cause life and health to abound as each stage of growth progresses. Lord, I believe I am redeemed from pain in childbirth, so I ask You to prepare my body to deliver this child without pain and suffering. I declare whatever ligaments, tendons, or tissues need to stretch, they will stretch. Father, I speak to my body and to my baby—to every part, every organ, every system to function properly and perfectly, fully developed as You intended from the beginning. I declare health, wholeness, soundness, spirit, soul, and body. Lord, I praise You for **supernatural childbirth**!*

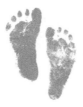

20-WEEK ULTRASOUND

Date of ultrasound: _____

Hospital/clinic: _____

Estimated due date: _____

Attach ultrasound picture

20-Week Ultrasound

Heart rate

_____

Length

_____

Weight

_____

Sex

_____

My thoughts as I saw my baby:

_____

_____

_____

_____

_____

_____

SUPERNATURAL CHILDBIRTH 40-WEEK PREGNANCY JOURNAL

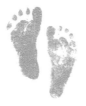

21 WEEKS PREGNANT

- Today's date: _____

- My current weight: _____

- My belly measurement: _____

- My scripture focus:

_____
_____
_____
_____
_____
_____
_____
_____
_____
_____

SUPERNATURAL CHILDBIRTH 40-WEEK PREGNANCY JOURNAL

- What I'm thinking and feeling most at this milestone of my pregnancy!

_____
_____
_____
_____
_____
_____
_____
_____
_____

Attach photo or memento here

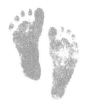

MY PRAYER FOCUS AND FAITH CONFESSION

And now, saith the Lord that formed me from the womb to be his servant (Isaiah 49:5).

Father, I come to You in Jesus' name with gratitude and appreciation. You bless the fruit of my womb. My child is fearfully and wonderfully made. Every day, Your Word is at work directing and guiding the formation of every muscle, organ, and system in my child's body. Because of Your hand upon us, my baby is whole and healthy. You have created this baby for greatness! Thank You, Lord, for the future You've planned for my baby. You have created in him/her all the specific talents, abilities, and traits needed to fulfill Your plan. I declare that my child will be taught of the Lord, and great shall be his/her peace. I will train this baby in the way he/she should go, and he/she will not depart. Lord, I ask You for the wisdom to nurture this child with the light to walk in Your plan and purpose. I believe You will equip me with every physical and spiritual provision I need.

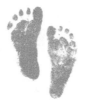

22 WEEKS PREGNANT

- Today's date: _____

- My current weight: _____

- My belly measurement: _____

- My scripture focus:

_____
_____
_____
_____
_____
_____
_____
_____
_____
_____

22 Weeks Pregnant

- What I'm thinking and feeling most at this milestone of my pregnancy!

_____
_____
_____
_____
_____
_____
_____
_____
_____

Attach photo or memento here

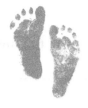

MY PRAYER FOCUS AND FAITH CONFESSION

Before I formed thee in the belly I knew thee; and before thou camest forth out of the womb I sanctified thee, and I ordained thee a prophet unto the nations (Jeremiah 1:5).

Heavenly Father, I am so thankful for the plan You have for my child. You have perfectly designed my baby with everything needed to fulfill the destiny You have prepared. In the name of Jesus, I pray for the path my child will walk to be flooded with light and protected by Your covenant. According to Psalm 37:23, let the steps my child will take be ordered by the Lord. Lord, guide him/her with Your laws (Ps. 119:133 TLB). Lord, show my child the path of life and hide them in the secret of Your presence (Ps. 16:11; Ps. 31:20). According to Isaiah 41:10, You will be with my child to strengthen and uphold him/her. Set the right people on that path to steer my child in Your direction. Give my husband and me wisdom to make decisions and provide guidance that will keep this child on track with Your best.

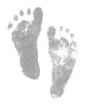

23 WEEKS PREGNANT

- Today's date: _____

- My current weight: _____

- My belly measurement: _____

- My scripture focus:

_____
_____
_____
_____
_____
_____
_____
_____
_____
_____

Supernatural Childbirth 40-Week Pregnancy Journal

- What I'm thinking and feeling most at this milestone of my pregnancy!

_____

_____

_____

_____

_____

_____

_____

_____

Attach photo or memento here

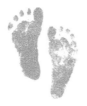

MY PRAYER FOCUS AND FAITH CONFESSION

After all, God is the one who gave life to each of us before we were born (Job 31:15 CEV).

Father, I thank You that You have blessed me with the baby in my womb. You are the Father of Spirits (Heb. 12:9), and the fact that You have given me this child in my womb is priceless to me. You have covered my baby in my womb (Ps. 139:13). I declare according to 2 Thessalonians 3:3 (AMPC) that the Lord is faithful and will strengthen me and the baby in my womb; God will set us on a firm foundation and guard us from the evil one. I decree, according to Psalm 121:5-8 (AMPC), the Lord is our keeper and the shade on our right hand. The sun shall not smite us by day, nor the moon by night. The Lord will keep me and my baby from all evil; He will keep our lives. The Lord will keep our going out and coming in from this time forth and forevermore. Father, I praise You for Your abundant goodness, in Jesus' name.

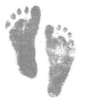

24 WEEKS PREGNANT

- Today's date: _____

- My current weight: _____

- My belly measurement: _____

- My scripture focus:

_____
_____
_____
_____
_____
_____
_____
_____
_____

24 Weeks Pregnant

- What I'm thinking and feeling most at this milestone of my pregnancy!

_____
_____
_____
_____
_____
_____
_____
_____
_____

Attach photo or memento here

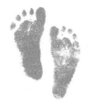

MY PRAYER FOCUS AND FAITH CONFESSION

But when it pleased God, who separated me from my mother's womb (Galatians 1:15).

I lift my hands and rejoice as I acknowledge that You are the one who will separate my child from my womb and escort my baby into my arms. I renew my mind to what Your Word says about birth and set aside every preconceived notion that comes from what society tells me about childbirth, and I dismiss any previous experience I've had. From this point forward, I submit to what Jesus provided for me in the work of redemption—freedom from the curse. I submit to Deuteronomy 7:13, which says You will love me, bless me, and bless the fruit of my womb. Lord, You said You take away from me all sickness (Deut. 7:15; Ex. 23: 25), and You make me a joyful mother of children (Ps. 113:9). Children are a heritage of the Lord and the fruit of the womb is Your reward (Ps. 127:3). In the name of Jesus, my pregnancy and **supernatural childbirth** *are submitted to Your plan, which is a plan to bless me! Thank You for Your supernatural provision and protection.*

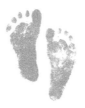

25 WEEKS PREGNANT

- Today's date: _____

- My current weight: _____

- My belly measurement: _____

- My scripture focus:

_____
_____
_____
_____
_____
_____
_____
_____
_____
_____

Supernatural Childbirth 40-Week Pregnancy Journal

- What I'm thinking and feeling most at this milestone of my pregnancy!

_____
_____
_____
_____
_____
_____
_____
_____
_____

Attach photo or memento here

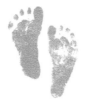

MY PRAYER FOCUS AND FAITH CONFESSION

And all thy children shall be taught of the Lord; and great shall be the peace of thy children (Isaiah 54:13).

*Heavenly Father, Your peace is a supernatural force that produces a life of **nothing missing** and **nothing broken**. According to Your Word, it is my heritage to have my children experience this life of peace and fullness. So, I rejoice that my baby is well and whole, with nothing missing in any area of their spirit, soul, and body. I speak Your life and peace to my child right now. I proclaim the peace of God to prevail in the bloodstream, in every organ, and in every bone. I speak peace to my child's immune system. I speak life to the muscles and tissues of my child's heart and brain. The peace of God is guarding my child and producing a life of nothing missing and nothing broken. Thank You for the wholeness and fullness of my child.*

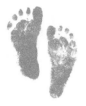

26 WEEKS PREGNANT

- Today's date: _____

- My current weight: _____

- My belly measurement: _____

- My scripture focus:

_____
_____
_____
_____
_____
_____
_____
_____
_____
_____

26 Weeks Pregnant

- What I'm thinking and feeling most at this milestone of my pregnancy!

_____
_____
_____
_____
_____
_____
_____
_____
_____

Attach photo or memento here

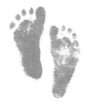

MY PRAYER FOCUS AND FAITH CONFESSION

Come to Me, all you who labor and are heavy-laden and overburdened, and I will cause you to rest. [I will ease and relieve and refresh your souls] (Matthew 11:28 AMPC).

What a benefit it is to have Your rest, Lord! I rejoice in the way Your Holy Spirit refreshes me every day in this supernatural pregnancy. I cast any and every burden, care, or anxiety on You! I won't worry about the natural preparations or the physical aspects of giving birth. As my body prepares for the delivery of my baby, my ligaments, tendons, muscles, and organs receive the necessary relief and refreshment for ease in childbirth. I speak peace and rest to the child in my womb. Father, I release Your rest and refreshing into my womb. I declare, according to Psalm 23:2 (AMPC), that the Lord leads us beside the still and restful waters. As my baby continues to grow and prepare for delivery, let every organ, muscle, bone, ligament, and tendon be strengthened and prepared for the days ahead.

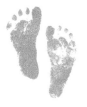

27 WEEKS PREGNANT

- Today's date: _____

- My current weight: _____

- My belly measurement: _____

- My scripture focus:

_____
_____
_____
_____
_____
_____
_____
_____
_____
_____

SUPERNATURAL CHILDBIRTH 40-WEEK PREGNANCY JOURNAL

- What I'm thinking and feeling most at this milestone of my pregnancy!

___

Attach photo or memento here

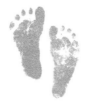

MY PRAYER FOCUS AND FAITH CONFESSION

Then [Ezra] told them, Go your way, eat the fat, drink the sweet drink, and send portions to him for whom nothing is prepared; for this day is holy to our Lord. And be not grieved and depressed, for the joy of the Lord is your strength and stronghold (Nehemiah 8:10 AMPC).

Father, Your joy is my strength and stronghold, so I stir myself up by rejoicing. Lord, I rejoice for Your provision of supernatural pregnancy. I praise You because You have redeemed me from pain and suffering in childbirth. I rejoice that You are my refuge and strength. I praise Your name that I am redeemed from a long, difficult labor, and I rejoice in the ease I will have in delivery. I rejoice in the health of my child. I yield to Your joy, knowing that it provides a spiritual strength. I want my spirit to be strong and full of joy because joy and peace work with my faith. Thank You, Lord, for the joy that provides a continual flow of strength to every area of my life.

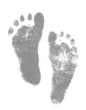

THIRD TRIMESTER CHECKLIST

So close!

- Schedule third trimester prenatal visits and tests
- Keep track of baby's movements
- Create birth plan
- Pack hospital bag
- Tour hospital or set up home birth
- Send baby shower "thank you" notes
- Prepare nursery
- Purchase and install car seat
- Choose your baby's name
- Pack diaper bag
- Stock up on household supplies

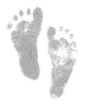

28 WEEKS PREGNANT

- Today's date: _____

- My current weight: _____

- My belly measurement: _____

- My scripture focus:

_____
_____
_____
_____
_____
_____
_____
_____
_____
_____
_____

- What I'm thinking and feeling most at this milestone of my pregnancy!

_____
_____
_____
_____
_____
_____
_____
_____
_____

Attach photo or memento here

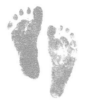

MY PRAYER FOCUS AND FAITH CONFESSION

But they that wait upon the Lord shall renew their strength; they shall mount up with wings as eagles; they shall run, and not be weary; and they shall walk, and not faint (Isaiah 40:31).

Father, as I walk through this last trimester, I walk in renewed strength. I will run and not be weary. I will walk and not faint. I declare Your supernatural strength flows through my being. According to Habakkuk 3:19, I declare the Lord God is my strength and He will make my feet like hinds' feet, and He will make me to walk upon mine high places. You are the God who gives strength and power to Your people (Ps. 68:35). I am strong in You, Lord, and the power of Your might. In the name of Jesus, I call my body strong. I speak strength to my womb, to my bloodstream, and to my heart. I confess Your strength to my baby. Let every part of my baby's body be alive with the strength and power of God. I praise You, Lord, for renewing my strength.

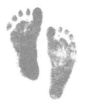

29 WEEKS PREGNANT

- Today's date: _____

- My current weight: _____

- My belly measurement: _____

- My scripture focus:

_____
_____
_____
_____
_____
_____
_____
_____
_____
_____

29 Weeks Pregnant

- What I'm thinking and feeling most at this milestone of my pregnancy!

_____
_____
_____
_____
_____
_____
_____
_____
_____

Attach photo or memento here

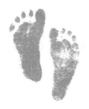

MY PRAYER FOCUS AND FAITH CONFESSION

Thou wilt keep him in perfect peace, whose mind is stayed on thee: because he trusteth in thee (Isaiah 26:3).

Heavenly Father, I choose to yield to Your peace by trusting in You. I will not fear or worry! In Jesus' name, I cast the cares of every decision and the preparations I need to make onto You because You care for me. Instead of being anxious about the financial responsibilities or preparations I need to make, I look to You. You will help me and give me the supply and wisdom I need. Lord, I will not worry about the day of my delivery. I refuse to allow anxiety to enter my heart about my labor or the delivery of my baby. I look to Your Word to strengthen my body to carry this baby to full term and provide all that my child needs to grow strong. I declare that You are my refuge and strong tower! I trust in You. I am submitted to Your Word! I depend on Your Word to provide the strength I need to deliver my child. Thank You for Your steadfast love for me and the baby in my womb!

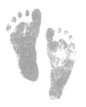

30 WEEKS PREGNANT

- Today's date: _____

- My current weight: _____

- My belly measurement: _____

- My scripture focus:

_____
_____
_____
_____
_____
_____
_____
_____
_____
_____

- What I'm thinking and feeling most at this milestone of my pregnancy!

Attach photo or memento here

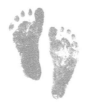

MY PRAYER FOCUS AND FAITH CONFESSION

That ye be not slothful, but followers of them who through faith and patience inherit the promises. For when God made promise to Abraham, because he could swear by no greater, he sware by himself, saying, Surely blessing I will bless thee, and multiplying I will multiply thee (Hebrews 6:12-14).

*Father, I put my confident trust in Your covenant promise to me. I am an heir of the blessing because I am Abraham's heir in Christ. Your blessing is the supernatural force governing my body, the baby in my womb, and even my delivery. In the name of Jesus, I stand on Your Word and inherit the blessing of **supernatural childbirth** and ease in delivery. I receive Your blessing and favor for the life of my child. Every day as my baby continues to grow, Your blessing dominates and guides the development of every organ and system in my child's body and Your favor ministers to my child's spirit.*

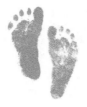

31 WEEKS PREGNANT

- Today's date: _____

- My current weight: _____

- My belly measurement: _____

- My scripture focus:

_____
_____
_____
_____
_____
_____
_____
_____
_____

31 Weeks Pregnant

- What I'm thinking and feeling most at this milestone of my pregnancy!

_____
_____
_____
_____
_____
_____
_____
_____
_____

Attach photo or memento here

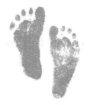

MY PRAYER FOCUS AND FAITH CONFESSION

For thou, Lord, wilt bless the righteous; with favour wilt thou compass him as with a shield (Psalm 5:12).

I choose to focus on Your favor, Lord. Your favor is around me like a shield! Not only does Your favor protect me, it causes Your goodness and blessing to prevail in every situation. Already, Your favor has supplied strength to my body during the past trimesters, helping me as my child has developed. Even now, Your favor is saturating my womb and ministering to my baby! In the days ahead, I will acknowledge Your favor is at work, and Your blessing is directing the course of my delivery. I declare, "The favor of God is governing my childbirth!" Thank You, Lord, for Your favor that surrounds me!

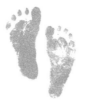

32 WEEKS PREGNANT

- Today's date: _____

- My current weight: _____

- My belly measurement: _____

- My scripture focus:

_____
_____
_____
_____
_____
_____
_____
_____
_____
_____
_____
_____
_____

Supernatural Childbirth 40-Week Pregnancy Journal

- What I'm thinking and feeling most at this milestone of my pregnancy!

_____
_____
_____
_____
_____
_____
_____
_____

Attach photo or memento here

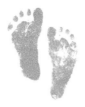

MY PRAYER FOCUS AND FAITH CONFESSION

For the Lord God is a Sun and Shield; the Lord bestows [present] grace and favor and [future] glory (honor, splendor, and heavenly bliss)! No good thing will He withhold from those who walk uprightly (Psalm 84:11 AMPC).

Heavenly Father, I am so grateful for the child You have formed in my womb. You are intimately acquainted with every detail of my baby's formation. Each day, Your blessing equips my immune system, my endocrine system, my bloodstream, and my womb so that my baby receives everything necessary to thrive. My whole body is flowing in the Spirit life of God. Thank You, Lord!

I speak to my body, "Be strong in the Lord and yield to the favor of God!" I set my expectations in agreement with Psalm 84:11, which says no good thing will God withhold from me. I expect every detail of my pregnancy to be marked with the goodness of God. I anticipate a pain-free and easy delivery, and I give You glory in advance! Praise the name of the Lord!

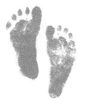

33 WEEKS PREGNANT

- Today's date: _____

- My current weight: _____

- My belly measurement: _____

- My scripture focus:

_____
_____
_____
_____
_____
_____
_____
_____
_____
_____
_____

33 Weeks Pregnant

- What I'm thinking and feeling most at this milestone of my pregnancy!

_____
_____
_____
_____
_____
_____
_____
_____

Attach photo or memento here

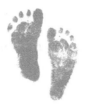

MY PRAYER FOCUS AND FAITH CONFESSION

I sought (inquired of) the Lord and required Him [of necessity and on the authority of His Word], and He heard me, and delivered me from all my fears (Psalm 34:4 AMPC).

*Lord, I am so grateful to You! Because I have You on my side, I don't have anything to fear. Instead, I trust in You. I choose to resist any thoughts that bring fear or anxiety about my pregnancy or delivery. I stand on the authority of Your Word against unrest or worrisome thoughts. I thank You for being my ever-present **help**!*

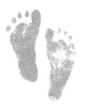

34 WEEKS PREGNANT

- Today's date: _____

- My current weight: _____

- My belly measurement: _____

- My scripture focus:

_____
_____
_____
_____
_____
_____
_____
_____
_____
_____
_____

SUPERNATURAL CHILDBIRTH 40-WEEK PREGNANCY JOURNAL

- What I'm thinking and feeling most at this milestone of my pregnancy!

_____
_____
_____
_____
_____
_____
_____
_____

Attach photo or memento here

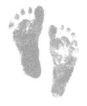

MY PRAYER FOCUS AND FAITH CONFESSION

O Lord of hosts, blessed (happy, fortunate, to be envied) is the man who trusts in You [leaning and believing on You, committing all and confidently looking to You, and that without fear or misgiving]! (Psalm 84:12 AMPC)

God, I trust in Your generous favor and blessing. Thank You for strengthening my baby within me and nourishing every organ and bone with health. I confidently look to You for Your supernatural power to flow through my bloodstream, administering the peace and joy of Your Spirit to every cell of my baby's body. In Jesus' name, I trust You to prepare my body for ease in childbirth and a quick delivery. Thank You for Your faithfulness!

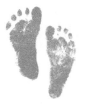

35 WEEKS PREGNANT

- Today's date: _____

- My current weight: _____

- My belly measurement: _____

- My scripture focus:

_____
_____
_____
_____
_____
_____
_____
_____
_____
_____
_____

35 Weeks Pregnant

- What I'm thinking and feeling most at this milestone of my pregnancy!

_____
_____
_____
_____
_____
_____
_____
_____
_____
_____

Attach photo or memento here

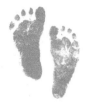

MY PRAYER FOCUS AND FAITH CONFESSION

For I know the thoughts that I think toward you, saith the Lord, thoughts of peace, and not of evil, to give you an expected end (Jeremiah 29:11).

As my delivery date approaches, I establish Your peace as the standard for the days ahead. You have provided me with a covenant of peace, and I rely on the protection and supernatural provision of that covenant. Your peace causes wholeness to flow into every aspect of this delivery. I declare Your peace will flood the atmosphere in the delivery room. Every nurse, doctor, midwife, and family member will be in the flow of Your peace. My thoughts and expectations are submitted to Your supernatural peace and joy! Thank You, Lord, for a peace-filled delivery.

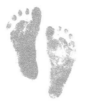

36 WEEKS PREGNANT

- Today's date: _____

- My current weight: _____

- My belly measurement: _____

- My scripture focus:

_____
_____
_____
_____
_____
_____
_____
_____
_____
_____

SUPERNATURAL CHILDBIRTH 40-WEEK PREGNANCY JOURNAL

- What I'm thinking and feeling most at this milestone of my pregnancy!

_____
_____
_____
_____
_____
_____
_____
_____
_____

Attach photo or memento here

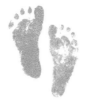

MY PRAYER FOCUS AND FAITH CONFESSION

Oh, how great is Your goodness, which You have laid up for those who fear, revere, and worship You, goodness which You have wrought for those who trust and take refuge in You before the sons of men! (Psalm 31:19 AMPC)

I celebrate Your goodness, Lord. It is Your goodness that has redeemed my pregnancy from the curse. Because Jesus Christ shed His blood, dying for me on the cross, I am free from the curse of having a long, painful delivery. Because of Your goodness, I am delivered from trouble and destruction! Thank You, Lord! Your goodness is supplying divine guidance and filling me with wisdom to raise my child in the nurture and admonition of the Lord. I declare today, "Jesus is made unto me wisdom" (1 Cor. 1:30). Thank You for that wisdom!

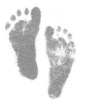

37 WEEKS PREGNANT

- Today's date: _____

- My current weight: _____

- My belly measurement: _____

- My scripture focus:

_____
_____
_____
_____
_____
_____
_____
_____
_____
_____

37 Weeks Pregnant

- What I'm thinking and feeling most at this milestone of my pregnancy!

_____
_____
_____
_____
_____
_____
_____
_____
_____

Attach photo or memento here

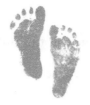

MY PRAYER FOCUS AND FAITH CONFESSION

Peace I leave with you, my peace I give unto you: not as the world giveth, give I unto you. Let not your heart be troubled, neither let it be afraid (John 14:27).

Today I declare, "Jesus Christ Himself has given me His peace. The peace of God protects my mind and heart from the entrance of worry or anxiety. I do not allow my heart to be troubled or afraid."

Lord, I keep my mind focused on You by holding fast to my confession of faith. Like You told Terry Mize to "mirror" Your Word to You, I hold Your Word up to You and repeat what You have said. You said that I am saved in childbirth (1 Tim. 2:15). You said that Christ has redeemed me from the curse of the law (Gal. 3:13). According to Psalm 103, I won't forget Your benefits. My iniquities are forgiven, and You redeem my life from destruction. You crown me with Your lovingkindness and tender mercies. Thank You, Lord, in Jesus' name!

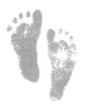

38 WEEKS PREGNANT

- Today's date: _____

- My current weight: _____

- My belly measurement: _____

- My scripture focus:

_____
_____
_____
_____
_____
_____
_____
_____
_____
_____

SUPERNATURAL CHILDBIRTH 40-WEEK PREGNANCY JOURNAL

- What I'm thinking and feeling most at this milestone of my pregnancy!

_____
_____
_____
_____
_____
_____
_____
_____

Attach photo or memento here

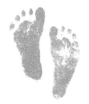

MY PRAYER FOCUS AND FAITH CONFESSION

Be careful for nothing; but in every thing by prayer and supplication with thanksgiving let your requests be made known unto God. And the peace of God, which passeth all understanding, shall keep your hearts and minds through Christ Jesus (Philippians 4:6-7).

*Lord, I will spend this week practicing Your peace. I refuse to be anxious. Instead, I yield to the protection of Your peace by declaring Your Word. Some trust in horses, some in chariots, but I trust in and boast of the name of the Lord my God (Ps. 20:7 AMPC). Lord, You are my refuge and my fortress. In You I trust. Surely You will deliver me from the snare of the fowler and the noisome pestilence. You shall cover me with Your feathers, and under Your wings, I will trust. No evil shall befall me or my child. Neither shall any plague come near our dwelling. For You shall give Your angels charge over us to keep us in all of our ways (Ps. 91). Thank You, Lord, for supernatural peace and **supernatural childbirth**!*

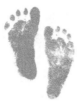

39 WEEKS PREGNANT

- Today's date: _____

- My current weight: _____

- My belly measurement: _____

- My scripture focus:

_____
_____
_____
_____
_____
_____
_____
_____
_____

39 Weeks Pregnant

- What I'm thinking and feeling most at this milestone of my pregnancy!

_____
_____
_____
_____
_____
_____
_____
_____
_____

Attach photo or memento here

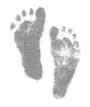

MY PRAYER FOCUS AND FAITH CONFESSION

The Lord is my rock, and my fortress, and my deliverer; my God, my strength, in whom I will trust; my buckler, and the horn of my salvation, and my high tower (Psalm 18:2).

I trust in You, Lord, with all of my heart. I rehearse Your Word and hold fast my confession of faith. As I look forward to delivery of my sweet baby, having enjoyed a blessed pregnancy of full duration, I thank You in advance for Your Word, Your blessings, Your peace, Your presence, and Your divine intervention. I pray and confess that my body and my baby will cooperate with perfect, supernatural delivery, that there will be no problems of any kind. I also believe and declare that my labor and delivery will be quick, short, easy, and painless. I believe and declare that I'll have time to get to the proper place with the proper help.

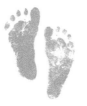

40 WEEKS PREGNANT

- Today's date: _____

- My current weight: _____

- My belly measurement: _____

- My scripture focus:

_____

_____

_____

_____

_____

_____

_____

_____

_____

_____

Supernatural Childbirth 40-Week Pregnancy Journal

- What I'm thinking and feeling most at this milestone of my pregnancy!

Attach photo or memento here

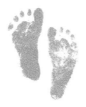

MY PRAYER FOCUS AND FAITH CONFESSION

I can do all things through Christ which strengtheneth me (Philippians 4:13).

Father, I believe that at the proper time for delivery, my water will break, and my uterus will do its job and begin to contract and push my baby down the birth canal. I command my cervix to dilate fully to 10 centimeters, to be elastic and stretch. I speak to my uterus, vagina, perineum, vulva, and cervix—you relax, be elastic and stretch without causing pain or any complications. Accommodate the birth of my baby. Furthermore, I declare in Jesus' name that I will not tear or need an episiotomy. Father, pain is under the curse of the Law, and Your Word says that Jesus bore our pain, so I rebuke all pain and will not tolerate pain. I will have a short, easy, pain-free delivery in Jesus' name; therefore, I won't need any anesthetic of any kind. Thank You, Lord, in Jesus' name.

I pray for the medical professionals who are involved with the birth of our baby, that they have the mind of Christ and wisdom of God concerning our family and this baby. The eyes of their understanding be opened that You, Father, lead and guide them how to care for us by Your Spirit. I say we have favor with them, that they are cooperative with us and what we are doing, that all is well and peaceful and under control in Jesus' name.

Baby, in Jesus' name, you move and place yourself in the perfect position for birth: head first, not breech, and face down. You rotate properly as God intended you to. I command the umbilical cord to be in the proper position as well. Body, you function perfectly during this time. I have perfect peace and am relaxed. All fear must go and stay gone, for I have God, who is perfect love and casts out fear. My body will not be tense but relaxed, at peace. In Jesus' name, **amen**!

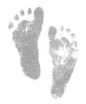

KEEPING TRACK OF MY BABY'S MOVEMENTS

Take time each day to track your baby's movements. Lay on your left side and note when your baby starts to move. Count each movement until you reach ten times and note that on your chart. You should be able to feel ten movements within the space of two hours.

Week 28 date: _____

	Start Time	Ten Kicks
Day 1	_____	_____
Day 2	_____	_____
Day 3	_____	_____
Day 4	_____	_____
Day 5	_____	_____
Day 6	_____	_____
Day 7	_____	_____

Week 29 date: _____

	Start Time	Ten Kicks
Day 1		
Day 2		
Day 3		
Day 4		
Day 5		
Day 6		
Day 7		

Week 30 date: _____

	Start Time	Ten Kicks
Day 1		
Day 2		
Day 3		
Day 4		
Day 5		
Day 6		
Day 7		

Keeping Track of My Baby's Movements

Week 31 date: _____

	Start Time	Ten Kicks
Day 1	_____	_____
Day 2	_____	_____
Day 3	_____	_____
Day 4	_____	_____
Day 5	_____	_____
Day 6	_____	_____
Day 7	_____	_____

Week 32 date: _____

	Start Time	Ten Kicks
Day 1	_____	_____
Day 2	_____	_____
Day 3	_____	_____
Day 4	_____	_____
Day 5	_____	_____
Day 6	_____	_____
Day 7	_____	_____

Week 33 date: _____

	Start Time	Ten Kicks
Day 1	_____	_____
Day 2	_____	_____
Day 3	_____	_____
Day 4	_____	_____
Day 5	_____	_____
Day 6	_____	_____
Day 7	_____	_____

Week 34 date: _____

	Start Time	Ten Kicks
Day 1	_____	_____
Day 2	_____	_____
Day 3	_____	_____
Day 4	_____	_____
Day 5	_____	_____
Day 6	_____	_____
Day 7	_____	_____

Keeping Track of My Baby's Movements

Week 35 date: _____

	Start Time	Ten Kicks
Day 1	_____	_____
Day 2	_____	_____
Day 3	_____	_____
Day 4	_____	_____
Day 5	_____	_____
Day 6	_____	_____
Day 7	_____	_____

Week 36 date: _____

	Start Time	Ten Kicks
Day 1	_____	_____
Day 2	_____	_____
Day 3	_____	_____
Day 4	_____	_____
Day 5	_____	_____
Day 6	_____	_____
Day 7	_____	_____

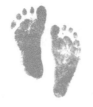

CHOOSING MY BABY'S NAME

Boy names	
Girl names	
Final choice	
Why I chose this name	

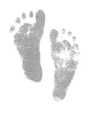

A LETTER TO MY BABY

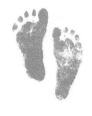

MY PRAYER FOR MY BABY'S FUTURE

_____
_____
_____
_____
_____
_____
_____
_____
_____
_____
_____
_____

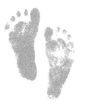

MY BABY SHOWER

Date: _____

Location: _____

Who attended

_____
_____
_____
_____
_____

Best moment

_____
_____
_____
_____
_____
_____

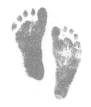

POSTPARTUM CHECKLIST

Let's Plan Ahead!

- Large maxi pads
- Large comfy pants
- Ice pack
- Witch hazel pads
- Epsom salts
- Stool softener
- Breast pads
- Pain reliever

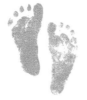

MY BIRTH PLAN

A birth plan provides a blueprint of how you envision your baby's delivery and helps you answer the important questions beforehand so you can communicate your preferences to those assisting you in this supernatural childbirth.

Name: _____

Expected due date: _____

Doctor/midwife: _____

Birthing place: _____

Support person(s) during labor and or birth:

Name:	Relationship:
Name:	Relationship:

Atmosphere

- Light dimmed
- Music
- Quiet with few interruptions

Equipment

- Birthing ball
- Birth stool
- Squat bar
- Tub
- _____
- _____

Birth Positions I Prefer

- In bed
- Standing
- Squatting
- Lying on side
- Kneeling
- Sitting
- Birth stool
- Birth ball

Labor

- I would like to move around freely.
- I would like to wear my own clothes.
- Fetal monitoring (continuous, intermittent)

My Birth Plan

- I prefer water to break naturally.
- Prefer during delivery (episiotomy or tearing)
- _____
- _____

During Delivery

- Mirror to view birth
- I would like coaching on when and how to push.
- Delivery planned as _____ (vaginal or C-section; water birth or Vbac)
- If C-section: (view birth if possible, arms free for skin-to-skin immediately, umbilical left to be cut by selected person)
- Support person present

Postpartum

- I plan to: _____ (breastfeed, formula, or combination).
- If a boy, I would like him to be circumcised: _____
- I would like to delay all procedures until skin-to-skin for 30 minutes/an hour.

Pain Management

- Offer medication when I appear to be in pain.
- Please do not offer pain medication unless I request it.

Supernatural Childbirth 40-Week Pregnancy Journal

- I'd like to use alternative pain control measures (breathing, massage, etc.).
- _____
- _____

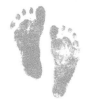

HOSPITAL BAG LIST

For Mommy

- Birth plan
- Wallet and ID
- Insurance card
- Hospital forms
- Going-home outfit
- Robe
- Gown or pajamas
- Nursing bra and pads
- Warm socks with grip or slippers
- Nipple cream
- Maxi pads
- Lip balm
- Glasses/contacts and solution
- Deodorant
- Makeup/toiletries

For Baby

- Going-home outfit
- Extra outfits
- Diapers
- Baby lotion
- Diaper cream
- Receiving blanket
- Burp cloths
- Car Seat

Extras

- Phone and charger
- Tablet/laptop
- Cash/coins for vending machine or parking
- Water bottle
- Headphones/earbuds
- Snacks and drinks
- Breast-feeding pillow
- Camera/video camera with memory card
- _____
- _____
- _____

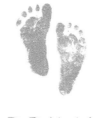

ARRIVAL!

Attach picture of here

Name: _____

Date: _____

Time of birth: _____

Place of birth: _____

Tell the story:

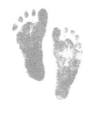

THE DETAILS

Time in labor: _____

Weight: _____

Length: _____

Sex: _____

Eye color: _____

Hair color: _____

Who cut the cord: _____

Doctor/midwife: _____

Who came to visit: _____

Seeing my baby for the first time: _____

Holding my baby for the first time: _____

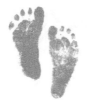

HOME SWEET HOME

Date

Attach picture of here

Where we live

Home Sweet Home

Who visited

_____

_____

_____

The first thing we did

_____

_____

_____

My memories of that day

_____

_____

_____

_____

_____

_____

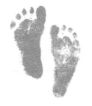

CONFESSIONS AND PRAYERS

From *Supernatural Childbirth: Experiencing the Promises of God Concerning Conception and Delivery*

Dealing with Fear and Thoughts

Fear is a spiritual force. It is the opposite of faith. Fear is real, and it is not of God. It affects the life we live on planet Earth. It affects the physical body. It can put a wrinkle in the skin, change the color of hair, make the heart beat fast or even stop. It has killed many people over the years. The Bible says in the last days men's hearts will fail them for fear (Luke 21:26). Fear motivates Satan as faith motivates God. Fear is Satan's tool as faith is God's.

You only fear the unknown or past bad experiences. Past failures bring future fears. Fear and faith don't operate together. Fear is your worst enemy when it's allowed to operate. It can be one of the greatest causes of pain during childbirth.

Now, don't get scared. I've got good news for you. Actually, the Word of God has good news for you. The Bible says in 1 John 4:18 that fear has torment but perfect love casts out fear. Now, God is love, the Bible says (1 John 4:16), and you've got God, so fear must go.

Second Timothy 1:7 says, *"For God hath not given us the spirit of fear; but of power, and of love, and of a sound mind."* You can conquer fear in Jesus' name with faith in God's Word. And Romans 10:17 says, *"So then faith cometh by hearing, and hearing by the word of God."*

Confessions and Prayers

All through the Bible God says, "Fear not." "Don't be afraid." Doesn't it make sense that when you are at peace, your body will be relaxed; it can stretch more, be more elastic? On the other hand, fear causes your body and muscles and nerves to tense up, to tighten. Jesus said, *"My peace I give unto you"* (John 14:27). Faith in God's Word brings peace.

F—alse
E—vidence
A—bout
R—eality

Prayer/Confession

Father, I come before You in the mighty name of Jesus and the covenant of blood, and I rebuke fear and doubt and unbelief. Your Word says You have not given me a spirit of fear but of love and power and a sound mind. Your Word also says that fear has torment but that perfect love casts out fear and God is love; and I've got God living big in me so fear and torment go far from me now, in Jesus' name. I trust in the Lord; I will not fear; I will not be afraid. I have the mind of Christ and the peace of God. My mind and body, as well as my spirit, are relaxed and at peace. I refuse to let my heart be troubled or afraid.

The Lord Most High is my light and my salvation, whom shall I fear? The Lord, El Shaddai, is the strength of my life, of whom shall I be afraid?

Body, I speak to you to be at peace, relax, rest. Muscles, nerves, be at peace. I rest in faith in God's Word and thank You, Father, for total and complete peace and confidence, in Jesus' name. Amen (Ps. 112:7; Isa. 41:10; Ps. 27:1; Isa. 54:17; John 14:27; 1 John 4:18; Phil. 4:7-8; Eph. 4:27; Isa. 26:3; 1 Peter 5:7).

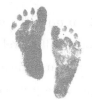

SCRIPTURES TO DEFEAT FEAR

When thou liest down, thou shalt not be afraid: yea, thou shalt lie down, and thy sleep shall be sweet (Proverbs 3:24).

I sought the Lord, and he heard me, and delivered me from all my fears (Psalm 34:4).

And to you who are troubled rest with us, when the Lord Jesus shall be revealed from heaven with his mighty angels (2 Thessalonians 1:7).

Casting down imaginations, and every high thing that exalteth itself against the knowledge of God, and bringing into captivity every thought to the obedience of Christ (2 Corinthians 10:5).

No weapon that is formed against thee shall prosper; and every tongue that shall rise against thee in judgment thou shalt condemn. This is the heritage of the servants of the Lord, and their righteousness is of me, saith the Lord (Isaiah 54:17).

He sent his word, and healed them, and delivered them from their destructions (Psalm 107:20).

Let us therefore come boldly unto the throne of grace, that we may obtain mercy, and find grace to help in time of need (Hebrews 4:16).

And be not conformed to this world: but be ye transformed by the renewing of your mind, that ye may prove what is that good, and acceptable, and perfect, will of God (Romans 12:2).

For I know the thoughts that I think toward you, saith the Lord, thoughts of peace, and not of evil, to give you an expected end (Jeremiah 29:11).

Delight thyself also in the Lord: and he shall give thee the desires of thine heart (Psalm 37:4).

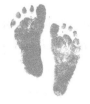

PSALM 91 CONFESSION

I don't know of a more effective confession in the Bible than Psalm 91. We confess this on a daily basis. The keys to making Psalm 91 work for you are found in verses 1 and 2. You must be dwelling in the secret place of the Most High, abiding in the shadow of the Almighty. How do you do that? Verse 2 tells you: You must, "Say of the Lord."

We pray it like this:

Father, we thank You that we (our family, our ministry) dwell in the secret place of the Most High, and we abide under the shadow of the Almighty. For we boldly say, decree, and declare that the Lord, El Shaddai, the God who is more than enough, Jehovah Jireh, Jehovah Rapha, Jehovah Tsidkenu, Jehovah Shalom, Jehovah Nissi, Jehovah Rapha, Jehovah Shammah, the possessor of heaven and earth, is our God. We trust in Him—some trust in horses, some in chariots, but we trust in the name of the Lord our God. He is our refuge and our fortress, our God, in Him do we trust. Surely He shall deliver us from the snare of the fowler and from the noisome pestilence. He shall cover us with His feathers, and under His wings shall we trust; His truth shall be our shield and buckler. We shall not be afraid for the terror by night, nor for the arrow that flieth by day, nor for the pestilence that walketh in darkness, nor for the destruction that wasteth at noonday. A thousand shall fall at our side and ten thousand at our right hand, but it shall not come nigh us. Only with our eyes shall we behold and see the reward of the wicked.

Because we have made the Lord, who is our refuge, even the Most High, our habitation, there shall no evil befall us, neither shall any plague come nigh our dwelling. For He

Psalm 91 Confession

shall give His angels charge over us, to keep us in all our ways. They shall bear us up in their hands lest we dash our foot against a stone. We shall tread upon the lion and the adder; the young lion and the dragon shall we trample underfoot.

We have set our love upon Him; therefore, He will deliver us. He will set us on high, because we have known His name. We shall call upon Him, and He will answer us. He will be with us in trouble; He will deliver us and honor us. With long life will He satisfy us and show us His salvation. Salvation is of the Lord. In Jesus' name (Ps. 91:1-16; Ps. 20:7).

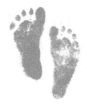

PSALM 103 CONFESSION

Father, according to Psalm 103, I say, "Bless the Lord, O my soul: and all that is within me, bless his holy name. Bless the Lord, O my soul, and forget not all his benefits." I say it and decree it over our family and our ministry and all that our family has anything to do with. I declare that those benefits belong to us. We'll not forget the benefits of the Lord: that our iniquities are forgiven, every sin is under the blood of Jesus. Father, Your Word says that if we confess our sins, You are faithful and just to forgive us our sins and to cleanse us from all unrighteousness. So we put every thought, every deed that's wrong, that is not pleasing to You, under the blood of Jesus. We ask for forgiveness, Lord. And we say that we are cleansed and forgiven in Jesus' name. Father, we thank You for that.

We say that You redeem our lives from destruction. We are protected by You, by Your Word, by Your angels. We'll not die prematurely; we'll not be destroyed. The destroyer, the accuser of the brethren, has been cast down. We're redeemed from destruction. Our lives will not be destroyed. You heal all our diseases. You crown us with lovingkindness and tender mercies. You satisfy our mouth with good things. I say that we have good things to speak and good things to eat so that our youth is renewed like the eagle's. We'll not be old, decrepit, and senile; even though we gain in age, we'll not go downhill. We wait on the Lord, and our youth is renewed.

Bless the Lord, O my soul, and all that is within me, bless His holy name. We thank You for all those benefits, and we'll be careful not to forget them. We give You glory and honor and thanks, in Jesus' name (Ps. 103:1-5; 1 John 1:9).

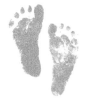

DURING PREGNANCY OR THREATENING MISCARRIAGE

You don't find "miscarriage" or "abortion" in the Bible. It was not and is not today the will of God for you to lose your baby. God wants you and your baby healthy, whole, and prosperous spiritually, physically, mentally, and financially. God is a good God.

There are multitudes of Scriptures you can pray and confess during this time, but these are good and will get you started. Use these Scriptures and the following prayer/confession all the time you are pregnant.

And ye shall serve the Lord your God, and he shall bless thy bread, and thy water; and I will take sickness away from the midst of thee. There shall nothing cast their young, nor be barren, in thy land: the number of thy days I will fulfil (Exodus 23:25-26).

And he will love thee, and bless thee, and multiply thee: he will also bless the fruit of thy womb, and the fruit of thy land, thy corn, and thy wine, and thine oil, the increase of thy kine, and the flocks of thy sheep, in the land which he sware unto thy fathers to give thee (Deuteronomy 7:13).

Bring ye all the tithes into the storehouse, that there may be meat in mine house, and prove me now herewith, saith the Lord of hosts, if I will not open you the windows of heaven, and pour you out a blessing, that there shall not be room enough to receive it. And I will rebuke the devourer for your sakes, and he shall not destroy the fruits of your ground; neither shall your vine cast her fruit before the time in the field (Malachi 3:10-11).

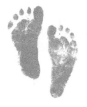

A PRAYER FOR BABY DEDICATION

We believe in presenting babies in solemn dedication to God. We see in the Bible that parents brought children to Jesus for His blessing (Matt. 19:13-15; Mark 10:13-16). Jesus put His hands on them and blessed them.

Hannah brought baby Samuel to church and presented him to God (1 Sam. 1:22-28). And Joseph and Mary brought baby Jesus to church and presented Him to God (Luke 2:22-24).

Terry and I, as ministers, have been brought babies by multitudes of parents and in some nations, we have not only had the job of dedicating the baby through prayer to God but of naming the child as well.

We have prayed over and dedicated our four children in formal church services with congregations as witnesses and also privately, both before conception and while the baby was in the womb.

Realize that "Baby Dedication" is your presentation of your child to God forever: that God be first and foremost in the child's life, that God use your child for His will, that God protect and provide for your child—spirit, soul, and body. You demonstrate the understanding that your child is God's and is only on loan to you, that you cannot just do as you please with your child but you have commandments and instructions in the Bible on how to rear and treat your child.

God said of Abraham, "I know him. He will command his children in the ways of God" (Gen. 18:19).

Remember, just because you give your baby back to God, He still expects and commands you to raise him or her and care for him or her on earth.

A Prayer for Baby Dedication

Here is a prayer you can adapt or pray as it is privately, just you and God, or before a minister in church.

Father, in Jesus' holy name, we come before You on this special day to present to You, to consecrate to You, to dedicate to You, to give back to You, this, our sweet baby that You have given us. Lord, we realize that we are only stewards of this special gift from You. Only You create life. This baby is Your baby. You said I must teach my children of You and Your commandments. You promised that if we would train up our child in the way he should go, he would not depart from it when he is old. You promised that if children would honor their parents, it would be well with them (not sick but well) and they would live long on the earth. You said they would be disciples of the Lord, taught and obedient to the Lord and great would be their peace and undisturbed composure. Thank You for these promises and commandments. Thank You for our baby.

This day, before You and the host of heaven and all other witnesses, we come to present to You in solemn dedication our baby. We consecrate as parents to not provoke him to wrath, but to bring him up in the nurture and admonition of the Lord. We commit to You to train him up in Your ways and he won't depart from them. We promise to teach him of You, Your ways, Your Word, Your will. We promise to train him by example and demonstration as well as our words. We promise to discipline him according to Your Word. We promise to love and care for him and bathe him in prayer from this day forward. We commit this baby into Your care. You are omnipresent; I can't always be there, but You can. Your angels have charge over him to keep him in all his ways and lift him up lest he dash his foot against a stone. We pray that this child be healthy, whole, complete, blessed, and prosperous spirit, soul, and body. We bind the forces of hell and the devil in Jesus' name to stay away from our family in every area of our lives. We decree that Jesus be enthroned above all else in our family at all times in Jesus' name. Amen (Deut. 6:6-7; Prov. 22:6; Eph. 6:1-3; Isa. 54:13; Eph. 6:4; Prov. 22:15; Prov. 29:15; Ps. 91).

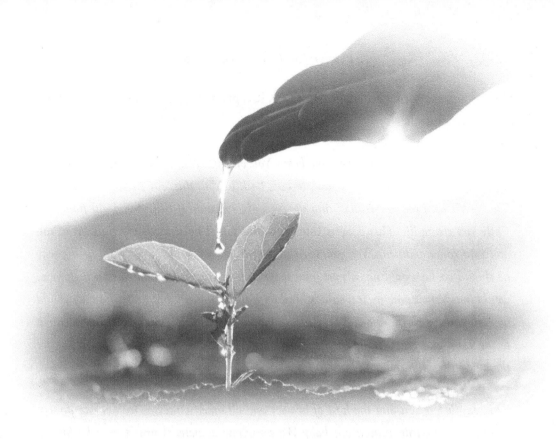

In the Right Hands, This Book Will Change Lives!

Most of the people who need this message will not be looking for this book. To change their lives, you need to **put a copy of this book in their hands.**

Our ministry is constantly seeking methods to find the people who need this anointed message to change their lives. **Will you help us reach these people?**

Extend this ministry by sowing three, five, ten, or *even more* books today and change people's lives for the better! Your generosity will be part of catalyzing the Great Awakening that many have been prophesying and praying for.

YOUR HOUSE OF
FAITH

Sign up for a FREE subscription to the Harrison House digital magazine and get excellent content delivered directly to your inbox!

harrisonhouse.com/signup

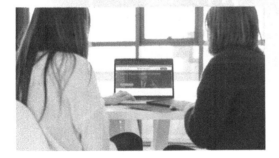

Sign up for Messages that Equip You to Walk in the Abundant Life

- Receive biblically sound and Spirit-filled encouragement to focus on and maintain your faith
- Grow in faith through biblical teachings, prayers, and other spiritual insights
- Connect with a community of believers who share your values and beliefs

Experience Fresh Teachings and Inspiration to Build Your Faith

- Deepen your understanding of God's purpose for your life
- Stay connected and inspired on your faith journey
- Learn how to grow spiritually in your walk with God

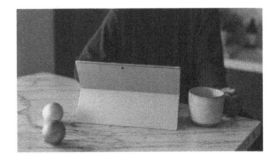

Check out
our **Harrison House**
bestsellers page at
harrisonhouse.com/bestsellers

for fresh,
faith-building messages
that will equip you
to walk in the
abundant life.